Tr

Susan Backhouse has suffered from IBS for several years and is co-founder of the IBS Network, a self-help group for sufferers. She is also the editor of the Network's journal, *Gut Reaction*. **Christine P. Dancey** is Senior Lecturer in Psychology at the University of East London and writes regularly for scientific journals. Their previous book, *Overcoming IBS*, was published by Robinson in 1993.

TREATING IBS

*Edited by Susan Backhouse
and Christine P. Dancey*

ROBINSON
London

Robinson Publishing Ltd
7 Kensington Church Court
London W8 4SP

First published in Great Britain
by Robinson Publishing Ltd 1995

A copy of the British Library Cataloguing in
Publication Data is available from the British Library.

ISBN 1-85487-314-8

Note
This book is not a substitute for your doctor's or health
professional's advice, and the publishers and author
cannot accept liability for any injury or loss to any
person acting or refraining from action as a result of
the material in this book. Before commencing any
health treatment, always consult your doctor.

Printed and bound in the EC

*Christine would like to dedicate this book to the memory of
Michael Davey (15.6.61–4.3.94) – love, as always.*

*Sue would like to dedicate this book to
Louise Maxey, with love and friendship.*

Contents

Acknowledgements

We are grateful to the Neal's Yard Bakery Co-operative for permission to reproduce the following recipes from *The Neal's Yard Bakery Wholefood Cookbook* by Rachel Haigh: hummus, gluten-free muesli, guacamole, Caribbean stew, swede and orange pie, strawberry mousse and dairy-free mayonnaise. We are also grateful to Rider Books for permission to reproduce the recipe for aubergine pie from *Greek Vegetarian Cookery* by Jack Santa Maria; to the Henry Doubleday Research Association for permission to reproduce recipes from *Good Food, Gluten Free* by Hilda Cherry Hills; to Berrydales for permission to use the recipe for chocolate cake from their newsletter; to the Ashgrove Press for permission to use the recipes for tofu burgers, brown rice digestive biscuits, potato shortbread and mock cream from *The Foodwatch Alternative Cookbook* by Honor J. Campbell; and to J.M. Dent & Sons for permission to use the recipes for millet and peanut cookies and carob fudge from *The Cranks Recipe Book* by David Canter, Kay Canter and Daphne Swann.

A Note on the Contributors

SUSAN BACKHOUSE co-founded the self-help organization, the IBS Network, and is the editor of its journal, *Gut Reaction*. She has written articles about Irritable Bowel Syndrome and, together with Christine Dancey, wrote the self-help manual *Overcoming IBS* (1993).

CHRISTINE P. DANCEY is Senior Lecturer in Psychology at the University of East London. Her research is concerned with the psychological effects of living with chronic disorders such as IBS, and she has published work (some in collaboration with Susan Backhouse) in scientific journals. She is co-founder of the IBS Network.

NICK READ is Professor of Gastrointestinal Physiology and Nutrition at the University of Sheffield. He has been seeing patients with Irritable Bowel Syndrome in a specialist capacity for over twenty years and has published three books and over three hundred papers on the condition. His career, developing through medicine, physiology, nutrition and latterly psychotherapy, provides a broad base for the development of more holistic concepts of understanding and treating IBS.

CLAIRE RUTTER graduated from The University of East London with BSc (Hons) Psychology in July 1994. In

September 1994 she started work as a research assistant, investigating the psychological effects of living with IBS in childhood.

ALAN STEWART qualified as a doctor in 1976. For the last twelve years he has specialized in nutritional medicine and is actively involved in teaching other doctors on the subject of nutrition. He has published widely on nutrition.

MARYON STEWART studied preventative dentistry and nutrition and worked as a counsellor with nutritional doctors for four years. She founded the Women's Nutritional Advisory Service in 1987. She has written several books on nutrition, including, together with Dr Alan Stewart, *Beat IBS Through Diet* (1994).

ELIZABETH E. TAYLOR has been using hypnotherapy and psychotherapy for ten years and has specialized in treating people with gut disorders for the past eight years. She worked alongside Dr Peter Whorwell of Manchester's Withington Hospital for three years. She is the founder of the Register of Approved Gastrointestinal Psychotherapists and Hypnotherapists.

BRENDA TONER is currently head of the Women's Mental Health Research Programme at the Clarke Institute of Psychiatry and Associate Professor at the University of Toronto. Her research interests include psychosocial assessment and treatment of Irritable Bowel Syndrome; and gender issues in functional gastrointestinal disorders. At present she is completing a randomized treatment outcome study on cognitive–behavioural group therapy for IBS. The treatment manual used in this study has been incorporated into a book by Drs Toner, Segal, Emmott and Myran, entitled *Functional Gastrointestinal Disorders: A Cognitive–Behavioural Perspective*, (1994).

Foreword

by Professor David L. Wingate

This is an unusual and welcome addition to the small but growing number of publications designed to help patients to live with the Irritable Bowel Syndrome (IBS). While IBS is a common condition, the pool of available advice is still small because the core of generally agreed data on IBS remains limited.

Not only is IBS a source of discomfort and distress to many thousands of people, it also defines an area of conflict between patients and physicians. Why should this be? The answer probably lies in the fact that the disorder is a constellation of symptoms lacking an agreed and objective pathophysiology. In most medical conditions, the dialogue between the patient and physician follows an accepted sequence. The first step is the patient describing his or her complaint to the physician. The next three stages consist of the discovery of physical abnormalities by the physician, the confirmation of the diagnosis by clinical or laboratory tests and, finally, the initiation of relevant treatment. In IBS, the last three steps are absent. A doctor examining a patient with IBS will find no consistent physical changes. There are no accepted diagnostic tests. Finally, there is no therapy that is accepted as effective in even the majority of cases.

Because only the first step in the medical process is present, IBS is the source of much frustration between patients and doctors. The patient describes the symptoms to the physician and awaits a response; often, there is virtually none, because, while the physician agrees with the diagnosis (which is often already known to the patient), there seems to be nothing more to be done. Patients are frustrated by what seems to be the inertia or even indifference of physicians, while physicians are irritated by the reiteration of complaints that sometimes sound trivial.

For all these reasons, IBS is a condition that is often marked by a poor doctor–patient relationship. This is why this book is so welcome. First, while the contributors are experts, as in many publications designed to help patients, they have been selected because they are individuals who have a positive approach to IBS and because they are able to suggest effective therapeutic strategies. Secondly, the editors have not been afraid of combining orthodox and alternative medicine between the same covers. Many patients and physicians are well aware of the potential benefits of a holistic approach to IBS that includes modalities such as nutrition and hypnosis, but books inspired by medical professionals have hitherto fought shy of explicitly acknowledging so much. This book is clearly designed to remedy that situation.

Susan Backhouse and Christine Dancey have already done much for IBS patients in Great Britain by setting up an active self-help network and this book is another welcome initiative from them. But it is not only patients who can benefit from *Treating IBS*; health-care professionals who want to understand what is important to patients in this field will be able to learn much from this book. It deserves to be widely read by patients and therapists alike. I wish it every success.

IBS: A Profile of an Invisible Chronic Illness

Susan Backhouse and Christine P. Dancey

What is IBS?

Irritable Bowel Syndrome is a disorder of the digestive system. We say 'disorder' rather than 'disease' because in this condition there appears to be no one part of the digestive system which is diseased or malfunctioning; rather, the system as a whole does not function properly. No hospital tests, X-rays or probes will actually find something 'wrong' in your system; they are undertaken so that other conditions may be ruled out. A condition like this is called a 'functional disorder'.

Although there is nothing diseased in the system, this disorder (as you will know only too well if you are a sufferer) can cause abdominal pain, diarrhoea or constipation (or an alternation of both), an urgent need to dash to the loo and numerous rumblings and grumblings in the digestive system (burbulence), along with flatulence, wind and bloating. Other symptoms that can be experienced include faecal incontinence, nausea, a sharp pain low down in the rectum and fatigue. These symptoms can be painful, exhausting, embarrassing and worrying.

Irritable Bowel Syndrome is one of several disorders grouped under the term Invisible Chronic Illness (ICI) by Drs Donoghue and Siegel in their book aptly titled *Sick and Tired of Feeling Sick and Tired*.* Other Invisible Chronic

* Details of this and other books mentioned in the text are given in the section on 'Useful Books' in the Appendix.

Illnesses include Lupus Erythematosus (lupus), lyme disease, migraine headaches and thyroid disease, and Irritable Bowel Syndrome shares certain characteristics with these other ICIs – pain, fatigue, bladder urgency, constipation, diarrhoea and sleep disorders, among others.

People with IBS, like sufferers from other ICIs, also often experience anxiety and depression. Most do not, as some doctors would have it, suffer psychosomatically from IBS *because* they are depressed, anxious people, but become depressed and anxious because they have a distressing condition which has no known cause and no cure, and who often receive little understanding from the medical profession.

What Happens to People with IBS?

Statistics tell us that a third of the population suffer from IBS at some time or another, and about 15 per cent have it seriously enough to cause them to consult their doctor. In fact, half of all visits to gastroenterologists are made up of people with function bowel disorders – many of whom have IBS. It's difficult to know whether the condition is getting more common, or whether it is simply being brought out into the open more.

Most people have experienced bowel symptoms at some time or another. Which of us can say we've never felt our stomach churn, or had an urgent need to dash to the loo just before something important or worrying? Also, digestive upset often comes after dietary indiscretion – many westerners find a bout of diarrhoea follows a meal of unusually hot, spicy food. And it is common to find that your bowels shut down for up to seventy-two hours after an abdominal operation or childbirth. No one worries about these symptoms if they occur infrequently – it is significant that in these instances you can understand *why* you've got the symptoms; you know that they are going to be temporary, and that you will soon be back to your usual self, when you scarcely notice what your digestive system is up to.

IBS and Your GP

However, you may be someone who suffers bowel symptoms more regularly. What was once a temporary set of symptoms may become more frequent, or more severe. Some people find that eventually they have some symptoms most days, and instead of being temporary, it just goes on, and on, and on . . . Eventually they go to their GP, hoping the doctor will be able to give them some medication which will bring them back to normal. If this has happened (or is happening) to you, or to someone you know, this story will probably be familiar to you. Your doctor tells you to take things easy and to come back in three or four weeks if the pain is still there. You may be given painkillers and/or medication for diarrhoea or constipation, and be told to keep to a high-fibre diet (not always the best idea; evidence shows this makes some sufferers worse: one study found that over 80 per cent of sufferers taking part had been prescribed a high-fibre diet but only 10 per cent were still following it, presumably because it hadn't helped them with their symptoms).

Both doctor and patient can become frustrated when the symptoms remain or are relieved only temporarily. Diana was told by a specialist that her chronic diarrhoea was the result of eating a 'typical western diet', low in fibre and with too many refined carbohydrates.

'He advised me to eat more wholemeal bread and cabbage. I was dumbfounded because he had come to this conclusion without asking me any questions about what I ate. As it happened, I'd been living on a smallholding. The large vegetable patch, soft-fruit garden, orchard and fields edged with blackberry bushes had given me ample supplies of fruit and vegetables, and I had regularly made my own bread with wholemeal or wheatmeal flour.

'Once [my GP] prescribed aspirin because it has a constipating effect. When I refused, he persisted and wrote out the prescriptions in spite of my protests. Tearfully, I tore up the prescription in front of him! I realized then that I had lost my faith in the medical profession.'

You may be told to slow down, avoid stress. But your symptoms don't go away. The medication may relieve some of the symptoms, but the remaining ones are often embarrassing; you don't like to tell people why you suddenly have to dash to the loo, or cancel engagements at the last minute. And so . . . you go back to your GP.

Hospital Tests

Although your doctor has heard that IBS can be diagnosed on the basis of symptoms alone, s/he is cautious; – s/he realizes that these symptoms could be due to other more serious diseases, such as colitis or Crohn's Disease. So just in case, you are sent for hospital tests; barium meal and barium enema, and maybe even a colonoscopy.*

All these visits to and from the doctor's surgery and waiting for hospital appointments take some months, months in which you may well feel anxious: you are not certain what you have, you probably don't know of anyone else with these symptoms, and you may also be worried that people will think you are malingering.

The tests turn out to be negative. The diagnosis: IBS. Although you should be pleased to discover you haven't got cancer, diverticulosis, colitis or Crohn's Disease you feel that the diagnosis of IBS is unsatisfactory, because you've read that there are no known causes, and no cures. You think: 'Why me? And why at this particular time?' Your GP may be supportive, but can offer you no definitive answers. Although some doctors say 'It's stress' and others say 'It's your diet', the honest answer is 'We don't really know.' We believe that IBS is a catch-all term for a collection of symptoms which

---

* Colonoscopy is a technique where an instrument is inserted into the rectum and up through the bowel. The instrument relays pictures of the bowel back to a screen. The process is carried out under general or local anaesthetic.

can vary quite a bit between sufferers, and which may have different causes.

Problems with the Medical Profession

The medical profession's track record of treating IBS patients is not a good one. We know of one fifteen-year-old girl who in the mid-1970s went to her doctor complaining of IBS symptoms. He felt her abdomen briefly and prescribed Valium! She was very worried about addiction and not being able to manage without the drug and, fortunately, took very few of the tablets. Nowadays, twenty years on, there is more awareness among doctors and few of them, it is to be hoped, would blithely send a young woman down the tranquillizer road. There are, however, still many sufferers of IBS who are less than satisfied with the treatment received from their GPs and from specialists. We found that almost all of a sample of 148 sufferers said that medical treatment was inadequate.

When Mrs Collins began to suffer from feelings of fatigue and breathlessness, together with pains in her head and flutterings and bangings in her heart, she suspected that the cause was the codeine phosphate she had been prescribed for her IBS. She was sent for exhaustive testing which revealed no organic problem. The consultant, who had been sympathetic at first, became much less so and eventually sent her to a psychiatrist, thus, she felt, 'washing his hands of me'. She went on to say:

> 'During this time, several suggestions by my husband and myself to the consultant that the codeine phosphate might be to blame were brushed aside.'

Mrs Collins was sent, at her own request, to another hospital where she was pleased to find she was treated with understanding and courtesy.

> 'Almost immediately it was suggested to me that the codeine phosphate was the cause of my troubles, apart from the basic bowel problem, that is. I was told to stop

taking it and ask my GP to prescribe a more up-to-date alternative. He prescribed Lomotil.

'My extreme tiredness vanished within a few days. My heart symptoms settled down and I discovered what it was like to feel well again. I feel that two years of my life have been wasted.'

What Causes IBS?

It will probably turn out that IBS has several causes, rather like obesity, for instance. Becoming obese can be caused by many factors, of which overeating is only one; others include underactivity, certain medications, and hormonal problems such as having a low thyroxine level. Some people put on weight easily; others tend towards thinness. With IBS, as with obesity, there is most probably a physiological disposition or tendency to IBS, which could then be 'triggered' by different factors. Stress, certain foods, drugs, gastroenteritis, abdominal operations such as hysterectomy – all these may trigger IBS in people predisposed to it. So *your* IBS may be triggered by stress; another person may have been symptom-free until they underwent a particular operation.

Physiological Theories
Some people may have an inbuilt tendency towards IBS. For example, the gut has its own nervous system called the 'enteric nervous system' (some gastroenterologists call this the 'little brain') There is two-way communication between this system and your real brain (often called the 'big brain'). IBS could be due to a failure in the way this brain–gut relationship works. Another theory of this type is that some people have oversensitive bowel muscle – perhaps inherited, or perhaps acquired from, say, an attack of gastroenteritis. There also seems to be a connection between hysterectomy and subsequent IBS, and gall-bladder trouble and IBS. Another idea is that food intolerance or allergy could cause these symptoms.

Is There a Link with Abuse?

Two separate studies have found a link between functional bowel disorders and abuse. One, done at the Mayo Clinic in the United States in 1992, looked at 68 men and 149 women who attended a gastroenterology clinic for functional bowel disorders (which include IBS). Sixty-six patients (30 per cent) reported abuse. Of these, thirty-nine had been sexually abused, fifteen physically abused and twelve both. The researchers found that patients who had been sexually abused were over two and a half times more likely to have functional bowel disorders than those who hadn't.

The Way We Live Now

It is possible that IBS is an consequence of the way most of us live our lives now. Long ago, situations which were threatening to us were dealt with immediate reactions – fight or flight. Nowadays, we have to cope with many frightening, threatening and unnatural situations without fighting or running away. We can use our wits; but our bodies still prepare us for the physical options. Our bodies, which have evolved to serve efficiently a lifestyle we moved away from thousands of years ago, have not had a chance to adapt to the drastic changes that have taken place since, in what, in evolutionary terms, is a relatively short time. It is possible that many diseases from which humans suffer today are, at least in part, a result of this 'evolutionary lag', and IBS may be one of them. An urgent need to defecate, for example, is part of the mechanism by which our body alerts us to danger.

What Part Does Stress Play?

The most common assumption by laypeople – and some medics – is that IBS is a reaction to the stress of life events. Some think it is due to an inability to cope, either part of the sufferer's personality or a 'conversion' symptom – in other words, because you cannot cope with a bad marriage or major relationship, and find this difficult to deal with, you convert your problems into bodily symptoms, in this case

7

IBS. Certainly, sufferers often *do* suffer psychologically – they may be anxious and depressed, and research has found that some sufferers remember being under a lot of stress before the IBS started. The problem with these retrospective accounts, however, is that many people can recall a stressful episode if asked to do so, even if they are not suffering from any symptoms, and people who are ill have a tendency to look back to find 'causes' which can explain their illness. Also, if IBS sufferers are told again and again that IBS is a result of stress (and most articles on IBS and books written on it for the layperson include stress as a major factor), the repetition can be very convincing! It is clear that stress can aggravate any illness, not just IBS, and it may worsen already existing symptoms; whether or not it actually causes or triggers symptoms of irritable bowel when the sufferer is in remission is less clear.

Some sufferers have given up work, thinking it is work-related stress which is causing their IBS; this helps some people, but others feel that it hasn't made any difference to them. Some sufferers say that their symptoms worsen when they are under pressure. However, many others have gone to great lengths to reduce the stress in their lives, only to find that their symptoms remain – or, paradoxically, that they suffer badly during relatively stress-free periods. This is what Maureen, who is in her seventies, found:

> 'My life is very curtailed by this condition which is a great pity as, after a very stressful life, I have now reached much calmer waters, and it seems very perverse that I coped with the stress and then develop this stressful condition when my life has become so much freer. I could live a much fuller and more outgoing life were it not for this condition.'

All in the Mind?
Living with a chronic disorder for which the medical profession and others have little sympathy can lead to psychological problems. For instance, ulcerative colitis, a disease with a

definable pathology which causes diarrhoea, pain and general ill-health, may take some time to diagnose correctly, during which time sufferers may be told that their symptoms are a manifestation of stress, depression or anxiety. One patient, before a correct diagnosis of colitis was made, was told he had underlying worries. When the patient said that he was unaware of this, he was told that he was worrying about something although he did not know it (in *Colitis*, by Michael Kelly, 1992). Studies have been conducted which have shown that colitis patients have psychological problems; however, these also show that the problems tend to subside after correct treatment, suggesting that the disturbance results from the disease rather than the other way round.

This may well be the case for many IBS sufferers. Ascribing psychological causes to illnesses is not a trivial matter for people who are suffering with obvious physical symptoms. Attributing a psychological cause to a disorder has both advantages and disadvantages. If someone believes that stress has caused their disorder or illness, then the solution for preventing a recurrence and becoming healthy lies within themselves. For patients with irritable bowel, attributing their disorder to stress means that they feel that they can, or should be able to, control it. The disadvantage is that, if symptoms remain despite all strategies for reducing stress (and this is most likely), depression and anxiety can result. Of course, if stress really *does* cause, or trigger, IBS, then such knowledge must not be withheld from sufferers; however, it is the case that at present *this really is not known*. While there is no doubt that emotional and psychological well-being contributes to physical health, it is common to hear people with IBS cite the stresses they have been through without any worsening of their symptoms.

Attributing a chronic disorder to 'stress' puts the onus firmly on the patient to change and recover, and is often an easy answer for professionals to give when at a loss to know how to explain irritable bowel. Medical practitioners have been found to attribute illnesses to stress when there is no *apparent* organic cause for a patient's distress. One study by two psychologists cited several examples of the reversal of cause and effect by health-care professionals when searching for causes of illnesses: mulltiple sclerosis sufferers are often told their symptoms are psychological or psychosomatic, and their strange behaviours labelled as neurotic or malingering, as are sufferers with myalgic encephalomyelitis (ME), primary dysmenorrhoea, diabetes and even cancer (notice all these are ICIs). The researchers noted these views particularly affect women, often assumed by medical practitioners to be more likely to be neurotic. Sufferers from endometriosis (a gynaecological disease) take an average of eight years to be correctly diagnosed. During the course of their illness they suffer severe abdominal pain, and their bowels may be affected – having a bowel movement can be painful, and they may suffer from diarrhoea. Three per cent of these women have previously been diagnosed as having irritable bowel, but their symptoms tend to disappear once the endometriosis is treated.

Health-care workers can be very dismissive of patients when they think patients have nothing organically wrong with them. Patients with Irritable Bowel Syndrome, often believing themselves to be the cause of their own disorder, and having only a few minutes to discuss their problems with the doctor, may leave the surgery feeling more miserable and 'stressed' than ever. The debate as to whether IBS is caused by stress, or whether having to live with it causes the stress, will no doubt continue for some time to come.

How do People Cope with IBS?

Psychological Consequences

Sufferers who work generally try to pretend all is well – apart from bowels not being a subject which people tend to talk about, they fear it might affect their job prospects if it were known about. Sadly, this is sometimes true – some employers believe IBS is a malinger's disease. Some people suffer so badly that they have to give up work. In our study three years ago we found that 5 per cent of people we questioned were unable to work because of their symptoms; a survey carried out later by Gail Rees of South Bank University found that 8 per cent were not working due to IBS.

Travelling also presents problems for sufferers with moderate to severe problems: they need to find out where the toilets are before they travel (16 per cent of sufferers said they had experienced bowel incontinence at some time), and traffic jams can certainly lead to anxiety.

All these problems can lead to a non-existent social life, when in fact sufferers *need* a good social life in which they can feel 'normal' and in which they can both give and receive support from others. Overcoming IBS is being able to cope with the psychological problems that *result* from the disorder, as well as being able to obtain some relief of your symptoms by means of treatment.

Having an invisible illness for which no organic cause can be found means that psychological explanations are often offered. The psychological consequences of disorders in which people *look* reasonably well are detailed in the book by psychologists Donoghue and Siegel, *Sick and Tired of Feeling Sick and Tired*. Take self-doubt for example. Many IBS sufferers begin to wonder whether they are really ill; are they imagining the pain, would it get better with 'positive thought'? Validation, and a recognition of what they are having to live with, is extremely important for many people with IBS. Lack of it can be destructive. Sufferers may blame themselves for 'causing' their IBS and their self-esteem will suffer. They may feel as if they should be able to control their symptoms and may try hard to 'pull themselves together', only to find that their IBS remains and on top of this they also have to cope with negative feelings about themselves, or even depression.

In spite of the growing awareness about IBS, the devastating effect it can have on those who suffer from it is generally underestimated. Some sufferers say they have been overlooked for promotion because of the time they have had to take off from work, or because their condition has hindered them. Others feel unable to tell their employers that they suffer from IBS, which can cause extra strain. Some people report that they cannot consider certain jobs at all – we know of sufferers who would have liked to return to work after having children but cannot; who cannot take any job where toilets are not easily accessible; some who cannot work outdoors, and others who cannot work indoors! Some jobs are ruled out because the potential extra stress involved is seen as likely to aggravate symptoms.

Claudia had hopes of going on to university and getting a good job, but had to leave school early because of her IBS:

> 'I plucked up the courage to get a better job, but I had to be choosy. It had to be one where I was free to go to the loo without being too obvious. I worked in a building society. This was fine until I progressed to being a cashier – as soon as I had a customer and thousands of pounds waiting to be counted I was churning inside and physically almost sick trying to get through to the end of the transaction. I eventually left the building society with 'nerves'.

When people begin to lose self-esteem, they become uncertain about where to go next. Travelling, changing jobs or making any sort of arrangements becomes difficult when you don't know whether you are going to be well or not. We wrote about these effects in our previous book, *Overcoming IBS*, and Donoghue and Siegel also show that these psychological effects are not specific to IBS; they are a consequence of having a disorder which is painful, disruptive of normal life – and invisible.

Of course, many sufferers find that their symptoms *can* be controlled in such a way that they are not overwhelming. We have heard from many people saying that since they have read books on IBS, and joined the IBS Network, they feel that they are no longer isolated and alone. Here, two sufferers illustrate what it meant to them to read about other sufferers through the IBS Network's journal, *Gut Reaction*.

'When I started reading all the newsletters, I cried: What a relief, I'm not going mad, after all. I was sent to many hospital psychiatrists. I now know I wasn't crazy, just needed some good advice like the newsletters have given me. IBS has cost me my marriage, almost my job and has made me feel unloved and lonely. But since reading all the great newsletters, I'm pulling myself together. I'm someone slowly putting my life back together with the help of *Gut Reaction*.'

'I felt I was coping badly – then I read the book, *Overcoming IBS* by Christine Dancey and Susan Backhouse. So many other people feeling the same way, indeed many were worse than me. Many were using the same excuses I did to avoid socialising, anything other than admit to having a bowel problem. It can be a very isolating problem. However, I now accept that I have a medical disorder. I've stopped feeling guilty and ashamed and will admit to it. I still have IBS but I feel much more positive about the future.'

Just knowing that there are thousands, even millions of people coping with the same sort of problems as they were experiencing made them feel a little better. Also, accepting that you have IBS, rather than constantly fighting against it, can be a source of relief. Accept your limitations; know what you can and cannot do.

In *Overcoming IBS* we described ways in which you could overcome the physical and psychological effects of IBS on your life. For instance, we talked about anxiety that accompanies IBS – What about the future? How can I cope? Will this affect my job? Sufferers worry about panicking, about incontinence and pain, and about not being in control of their own body. They feel embarrassed about their symptoms, and often feel inadequate because they feel they should be able to cope better with their IBS.

Both men and women find that IBS affects sex and relationships. We know of extreme cases where sufferers have felt it has cost them their marriage, or an equally important relationship. Other people can feel so inhibited and embarrassed by their symptoms that they are unable to embark on close relationships at all. Sex lives can suffer, or be non-existent: in our study we found that nearly half of those taking part (46 per cent) said that IBS interfered with their sex lives. And it isn't only women who feel reluctant about intimacy. Henry, a single man in his thirties, said:

'It makes it difficult to develop relationships with the opposite sex – what girl would want to go out with a man who daren't go out of reach of the loo? How can I be open with them about it?'

And Steven, who is in his twenties, explains how he feels:

'I daren't have a girlfriend. I lack self-confidence in that I am dependent often on being near a toilet. I feel different, abnormal and frustrated in not being able to do what I want.'

These difficulties are the more painful given that the value of having support and understanding from those close to them is often emphasized by sufferers.

And yet, in spite of all this, IBS is still considered to be a trivial condition. Is this simply because it is not 'life-threatening'? What about 'quality of life-threatening'?

Lifestyle Changes
Something which stands out very strongly is how much IBS sufferers do themselves to attempt to alleviate their symptoms and help themselves cope with them. Many alter their patterns of behaviour in order to find a lifestyle which minimizes the impact IBS has on them. Looking at, and altering, their diet is one of the first steps people take when

trying to help themselves. It is common to find people embarking on elimination diets to try to discover whether they have any food intolerance. Restricted diets such as dairy-free and wheat- or gluten-free regimes are often adopted, at least for a trial period. Some people find relief; other don't. If the IBS Network's members are representative, IBS sufferers are noticeably aware about healthy eating. We found that 70 per cent were trying to ensure they ate a balanced diet with plenty of fruit and vegetables, and as little processed and junk food as possible.

Some of the other lifestyle changes sufferers have made include cutting down on commitments so as to leave more time for relaxation; trying to be less competitive, both at work and during leisure time – replacing aggressive, competitive pursuits with walking, relaxation, meditation, yoga, etc.; and trying to keep calm when stresses do arise. It is common to find that sufferers turn to complementary medicine when allopathic (mainstream western) medicine doesn't help them, and positive lifestyle changes are often encouraged by practitioners of these alternative approaches. Complementary medicine has been helpful for some people and not for others. (See Chapter 6 for more about this.)

Difference in Coping: Early Learning

It is clear that some sufferers find having IBS much harder to cope with than others. Some find it easy to be open about their problem, while others tell only one or two close friends or relatives, or even no one at all. For some people, having IBS hasn't affected their self-esteem one jot; others suffer acutely from embarrassment, shame and feelings of guilt. Putting the severity of symptoms on one side, the way a sufferer feels about having IBS is a crucial aspect of how they are able to cope.

Like many aspects of our behaviour, the feelings that will affect our ability to cope with a condition like IBS can often be traced back to our very early years. A lot of damage can be done to a child who is made to feel ashamed about his or

her natural bodily functions. It is extraordinary how something so universal and so essential as having a bowel movement has been distorted. We know of one child who was very
surprised to find out that the Queen had them! Psychologist
Dorothy Rowe believes that the way children are toilet
trained can have a great effect on their future bowel health:

> For many small children the most stressful, frightening
> time of their life is the months, or even years, of toilet
> training. Many parents get extremely distressed and angry
> when their child fails to be continent according to the
> parents' wishes . . . The most common letter I get is from
> mothers and grandmothers who are greatly distressed by
> the child's failure to be toilet trained. They describe scenes
> which from the toddler's point of view must be extremely
> frightening. They say things like, 'I'm at my wits' end' and
> 'I've tried bribing him and slapping him, but nothing
> works.' 'When will he learn to be clean?', they ask, without
> realizing that the toddler is learning something very well
> and that is that anything to do with his bowels is associated
> with fear, anger and punishment.
>
> Toddlers are often shown that their parents, indeed
> everyone, rejects them because they have made a mess.
> The whole point of toilet training is to be clean, which is
> control and organization, as against dirty, which is uncon-
> trolled and chaotic. No wonder most of us grow up with
> many anxieties about being acceptable and being clean.
>
> For many people with IBS the worst part is not the
> painful physical symptoms but the fear of being rejected
> and being dirty. Thus their worry about being rejected and
> being dirty create the stress which initiates and maintains
> the physical symptoms.

How can it have happened that a normal, natural bodily
function can arouse so many ambivalent feelings? It is an
indication of the dis-ease from which our society suffers.
Gastroenterologist Ken Heaton of the Bristol Royal Infirmary
says that as a culture we have 'demonized defecation': it

cannot be discussed in polite company, it isn't mentioned on television (except in cheap jokes), very few books have characters in them who go to the toilet or have bowel movements (though Raymond Briggs's books for children and adults are a welcome exception!). This all makes it very difficult for anyone who has a problem with defecation to discuss it without fear of ridicule or embarrassment. Heaton points out how this can make it extremely difficult for a doctor to find out exactly what a patient's problem is. Many people have trouble just finding the words to describe what their bowels are up to and misunderstandings can arise. He remembers:

> A retired headmaster, who should have been a model of precise speech, once said to me, 'Doctor, I have great difficulty doing anything serious with my insides.' After several questions, he admitted that what he meant was that he had to strain to defecate! Another patient, who was asked to write down his complaints, put down 'unco-operative activities of alimentary canal' when he meant diarrhoea!

Increased Public Awareness

Since we set up the IBS Network in 1991 there has been a distinct rise in public awareness of IBS. More articles in newspapers and magazines, pieces on the radio and television, and more publications on the condition have all helped those who suffer from it to realize there are millions of people in the UK alone in the same boat as them. Today, if you tell people you've got IBS, it is much more likely you will hear of other people who also suffer than it was even a few years ago. And with the development of the network of local IBS groups, it is IBS sufferers themselves who are pushing for better understanding from the medical profession, for more information about IBS and for effective treatment to be available to all who need it.

Effective Treatment of IBS

Is there any effective treatment? And if so, what is it? In *Overcoming IBS* we described the treatments available for IBS sufferers only briefly – in just one chapter, in fact. In a general book about IBS it was impossible to go into all the available treatments in depth. In editing and contributing to this new book we have attempted to present the major forms of treatment available today for IBS sufferers. We can say, however, that at the moment there is no 'cure' for IBS. The methods of treatment available may help significantly with management of the condition, but they don't guarantee that symptoms will disappear for ever. For many of us with IBS, effective treatment is something that continues to evade us.

In *Treating IBS* we look at the allopathic medical profession and beyond – into the realms of those who treat and have been treated by holistic medicine, by techniques which treat the mind and by dietary methods; and we look at the power of self-help groups. A couple of decades ago, most of these treatment methods would have been non-existent or extremely rare. Most of them have only recently begun to come into their own in Britain. We can look with hope to the future as these methods become more refined and new forms of treatment are discovered or reintroduced (some of the complementary disciplines have been around for thousands of years).

You will notice that the views expressed by the authors in this book differ widely. This is because, although we now know a lot about IBS, the way experts treat sufferers depends partly on their views about what causes the condition in the first place. And however much one expert is convinced that his or her views are the correct explanation, at present there is no consensus of opinion.

Information is power, so gather as much information about IBS as you can, and try to decide which is the best way for you to tackle your IBS. We hope this book helps you to do exactly that.

2

IBS: A Gastroenterologist's View of Treatment

Nick Read

Our approach to the treatment of Irritable Bowel Syndrome really depends on how we view it. Is it a disease like ulcerative colitis or cancer; something tangible that we can see and diagnose with confidence? Is it a syndrome, like breathlessness or indigestion: a bodily discomfort and disturbance which can be caused by many different though specific conditions? Or is it the gut reaction to the vicissitudes of fortune, a disturbance that is neither all in the gut nor all in the mind but involves both? If IBS were a disease, treatment would be easy. It would be like treating a duodenal ulcer with tablets that block acid secretion or combinations of specific antibiotics. But research over the last fifty years or more has not been able to identify a specific disease mechanism for the Irritable Bowel Syndrome. In the future somebody may discover a specific virus or bacterium that is responsible for the condition, like helicobacter in duodenal ulcer disease, but so far, despite looking very hard, medical scientists have not come up with anything like that. So, because Irritable Bowel Syndrome does not appear to be a specific disease, there is not a specific treatment for it.

Is IBS a Syndrome?

What if IBS is indeed a syndrome, a well-defined cluster of symptoms, easily recognizable, that could be induced by several different conditions? The model here would be some-thing like asthma, the combination of breathlessness, whee-ziness and airway obstruction which can be brought on by infection, allergies to pollen, cold air and emotional factors. The fact that the condition is called Irritable Bowel *Syndrome* indicates that this is the current view. Most doctors would regard it as a syndrome that comprises abdominal discomfort plus a disturbance of defecation which might be either diarrhoea or constipation, or a mixture of the two, and a few rather specific symptoms like a feeling of incomplete evacua-tion (wanting to go to the loo again after you have just been), lower abdominal pain relieved by defecation, passage of mucus and an urgent desire to defecate.

In recent years, there has been a determined effort on the part of some experts to define rigid criteria for the diagnosis, so that researchers throughout the world can be sure they are studying the same condition and different treatments can be tested on a single well-defined entity instead of a hotch-potch of differing conditions which are collected together and called IBS. The problem with this approach is that everybody who has IBS is different. The combination of symptoms experi-enced by one person with Irritable Bowel Syndrome may be quite distinct from those experienced by another patient. For example, the patient who suffers from frequent passage of sloppy stools associated with abdominal pain and the patient who suffers with abdominal bloating and constipation are both included under the category of Irritable Bowel Syn-drome. Furthermore, the condition encompasses a constel-lation of other symptoms such as headache, tiredness, breathlessness, frequent passage of urine, backache, leg pains, depression, anxiety and so on. In fact, some patients have so many bodily symptoms that it may be a matter of luck whether they come to the gastroenterologist and are diagnosed as having Irritable Bowel Syndrome or whether they go to, for example, the cardiologist and are investigated for chest pain.

It is all very difficult; but perhaps it may be helpful to hold on to the notion that symptoms like a frequent desire to defecate, pain relieved by defecation, feeling of incomplete evacuation, rectal mucus and recto-anal spasms, imply an irritability of the lower end of the gut. This suggests that we should focus on what might be causing sensitivity or irritability in this region.

A Complex of Different Diseases

I am often struck by the notion that if we were puzzling over IBS fifty years ago, the whole portmanteau of conditions that cause abdominal discomfort plus a disturbance of defecation would include diseases like coeliac disease, ulcerative colitis, Crohn's Disease and cancer of the colon – distinct conditions that are easily recognized and diagnosed by doctors these days. So out of the large 'cake' that we call IBS, we have been able to cut slices which represent specific diseases and diagnoses. Perhaps if we pay sufficiently careful attention to what our patients are telling us we may still be able to recognize specific subsets of Irritable Bowel Syndrome that would respond to specific treatment. The following examples illustrate some of the possibilities for specific treatment.

Bile Acid Malabsorption

Joyce's story
Ever since her husband had left her, Joyce had suffered with quite severe diarrhoea, needing to pass soft liquid motions up to twenty times a day. Joyce was not getting any maintenance from her husband and had had to take a part-time job to gain enough money to keep the family together. Going to work was a nightmare. Since Darren was born three years ago, Joyce had noticed that she could be incontinent of gas or liquid motions. Just to travel on the bus she had to wear pads and towels and always take two spare pairs of pants with her. Her boss had already complained about the time she spent out of the office in

the loo. She was prescribed Questran as granules, which she mixed with a drink and took half an hour before each meal, adjusting the dose with the size of the meal (two before a big meal like dinner, and one before a small meal). Within two days, the diarrhoea and incontinence had gone – in fact, she was a bit constipated; but she experienced instead quite severe griping abdominal pains.

In recent years, some patients with frequent passage of sloppy or watery stools and abdominal pain have been treated quite successfully with resins that bind bile acids. Bile acids are normal constituents of digestive secretions. They act rather like detergents to disperse fat, making it much easier and faster to digest and absorb, and most are normally reabsorbed at the lower end of the small intestine. The overactive gut of Irritable Bowel Syndrome can cause food and digestive secretions to pass down the small intestine much more rapidly than normal. As a result, a lot of the bile acids are not reabsorbed and go down into the colon where they cause irritation, resulting in diarrhoea. Treatment with the resin Questran (cholestyramine) can mop up the bile acids and stop this happening. Unfortunately, not very many people with IBS like Questran. Some dislike the texture and complain that it makes them feel sick; others, like Joyce, find that the cost of getting rid of the diarrhoea is the development of pain – as if her distress has to come out somewhere.

Urgency and Faecal Incontinence

Diarrhoea can be bad enough by itself, but when it is associated with incontinence it is a disaster. Joyce has struggled on with difficulty. Other people tell me that they can only go out if they have a map of all the toilets in Sheffield just in case . . . and since the council has been closing 'conveniences' to save money, they live as recluses, confined to their houses.

This problem affects women in particular and in most it is caused by damage to the muscles around the bottom during childbirth. Even if there is no actual tear into the anus, the stretching that occurs as the baby is born can damage the nerve going to the anal sphincter and cause weakness that can get worse with time. A lot of research is currently being directed at finding out whether changes in obstetric practice can prevent this distressing complication of childbirth. Pelvic floor or 'Kagel' exercises may help the pelvic muscles to recover some strength after childbirth, but will not be much use if the muscle is torn or badly stretched. The only recourse then is surgery: either direct repair of the torn muscle or a strengthing of the pelvic floor with the surgical equivalent of a 'darn' or, occasionally, a 'patch' or graft. Most surgeons, however, would try to subdue the irritable bowel first before contemplating pelvic surgery.

Lactose Intolerance

This, like bile acid malabsorption and obstetric injury, does not actually cause IBS, but it can certainly make it much worse. Treatment is simple: a determined reduction in consumption of milk or milk products that contain lactose.

Lactose is milk sugar. In babies, it is normally digested in the small intestine by lactase enzyme to glucose and galactose, which can then be absorbed into the body. Most populations in the world lose their lactase enzyme around the time of weaning. This means that when older children and adults drink milk, the lactose is not absorbed and goes down into the large intestine, where it is fermented by bacteria yielding large amounts of gas. Reputedly the gassiest person in the world, Mr Sutalf, who once passed wind 144 times a day, was deficient of lactase enzyme but drank milk.

Impaired digestion of lactose may not be too much of a problem for most people, but those with the sensitive and reactive bowels of IBS may suffer agonies of pain, bloating, gas and diarrhoea, and gain much relief from dietary restrictions.

Too Much Fibre

Sam's story

Sam is a fit, assertive 25-year-old. She believes in looking after her body. She attends aerobic classes five times a week and she is very careful about what she eats, preferring cereals and vegetables and lots of fruit. Sam was well until she became engaged to John, who plays rugby and enjoys a drink with his mates. Sam developed abdominal cramps and became constipated; she felt like she was full of gas and worried about her protruding tummy. She began to step up her exercise programme and take more cereal in her diet. At first she resisted the idea that she should cut down her fibre intake and eat a more balanced diet containing meat and eggs and cheese, but after a few weeks of trying this change in diet her symptoms were not so severe. She expressed considerable anxiety about her engagement and asked if there was anybody she could discuss it with.

Like lactose intolerance, and for the same reasons, the enthusiastic consumption of dietary fibre often makes the symptoms of IBS much worse. Fibre contains polysaccharides that cannot be digested in the small intestine but are fermented producing a lot of gas when they reach the colon. Ideas regarding the use of fibre in IBS have changed. In the heady days of 'fibre for all' in the early 1970s many doctors believed that IBS was a disease of fibre deficiency, condemning many patients to agonies of pain and bloating and the embarrassment of gas and diarrhoea. While it is true that fibre can be very helpful for some patients with constipation, it tends to make other symptoms worse. These days I tend to advise people with IBS to restrict their intake of fibre.

Bile acid malabsorption, lactase deficiency, obstetric injury and ingestion of too much fibre do not actually cause IBS, but they can make the symptoms much worse. At the moment, there does not seem to be any specific disease that can reliably be said to cause IBS, but there are a few candidates.

Candidiasis

Petra's story

Petra was cross. She announced her intentions as soon as she came in. '*I've got candida. I've eaten yoghurt until it's coming out of my ears. I've taken courses of antibiotics until they've made me puke. I've even had my colon washed out three times. You are my last hope!*' We started to talk. Rather rapidly, as if what she was saying was of no consequence, she told me about her mother abandoning the family when she was two, the sequence of minders, raped by her uncle at fifteen, an abortion at eighteen, a failed marriage . . . '*And I don't want you to say it's all in my mind. I want you to look at the bacteria in my colon.*' I said that I would be glad to work with her but I could only operate in a way that I believe was best for her. '*Oh, so unless I fit in with your mind set, you can't help me,*' she retorted and stormed out.

The notion that a significant proportion of IBS may be caused by candida has received some public support but there is no good scientific evidence to support it. In any case, the large amounts of oral fungicides that need to be given to eradicate candida from the body can be quite toxic and cause other symptoms. I am inclined to think that for most of the time this organism lives in close harmony with us and only gets out of control in sites other than the vagina or the mouth if our immune system is severely compromised. There is no evidence to suggest the immune system is severely compromised in Irritable Bowel Syndrome. I could be wrong, but I remain to be convinced that treatment regimes aimed at eradicating candida have any lasting benefit for IBS sufferers.

Rectal Mucosal Prolapse

Surgical treatment for IBS has received publicity recently with the news that Mr Bernard Palmer, a surgeon working in

Stevenage, has been treating patients with IBS by taking tucks in the lining of the rectum to remove the superfluous 'skin' that may cause difficulty in defecation. At first, Mr Palmer selected his patients rather carefully – they were people who suffered feelings of 'rectal dissatisfaction', wanting to go to the loo but being unable to go – but he has since found that his operation can help even those people who have central abdominal pain or even indigestion. Mr Palmer reported that about 80 per cent of the patients he had treated were free of symptoms three months after their treatment.

The patients that Mr Palmer originally selected sound as if they might have had a mild form of rectal prolapse, where the lining of the rectum may actually come down and block the outlet, so frustrating defecation. Rectal mucosal prolapse or, as it is sometimes called, 'solitary rectal ulcer syndrome', can be recognized by the patch of inflammation or even ulceration in the rectum when doctors have a look inside with a sigmoidoscope. Long-term follow-up is necessary in order to assess the true efficacy of Mr Palmer's treatment. Until that is established, we have to keep an open mind, though I do find it hard to believe that something as simple as redundant rectal mucosa can be responsible for the multiplicity of symptoms that is IBS. Surgery, especially when conducted by a listening, caring and charismatic exponent, is a powerful placebo, but if it works, we should not knock it too much.

Diverticular Disease

Some patients with IBS have had undergone surgical excision of the sigmoid colon, on the grounds that this region of the colon can appear on X-rays or motility recordings to be in spasm. I cannot think of any patient with IBS who has been cured by such treatment. Sigmoid resection, however, has been quite successful in some patients with diverticular disease, a condition where the hypertrophied muscle of the colon results in high pressures and forces out little pouches at weak points in the wall. Diverticular disease is a disease of ageing, but it has been suggested that patients with long-standing IBS may be more likely to get diverticular disease earlier than usual – on the grounds, I suppose, that a stressed-out colon is more likely to age more rapidly than one that has not been subject to the vicissitudes of life. I suspect that the association between the two may be that the presence of diverticular disease can produce many of the symptoms of IBS. IBS is not just a disease of the rectum or sigmoid colon; in most patients it seems to involve most regions of the gut and many other organs as well. For most people, IBS is a disease of the whole body.

Post-Gastroenteritis IBS

Ray's story
'I know exactly when it started. I had been fishing with some friends in Norfolk. We were coming back along the motorway and we stopped in this cafe for a meal. I chose the fish. I knew there was something wrong with it, but I was hungry and I ate it. The next day I came down with the most awful diarrhoea and vomiting. It lasted three days and I felt really awful. The funny thing was that the diarrhoea never really cleared up. It's now three years later and I can still go five times in the morning, but them Ketotifen tablets you gave me certainly make it much more bearable. I can even play a game of football now.'

Ray had post-gastroenteritis IBS. A biopsy of his rectum showed a lot of inflammatory cells. Our recent research at Sheffield has shown that about 30 per cent of people who have an attack of gastroenteritis go on to develop IBS. We have been interested to find out whether there is any particular factor that distinguishes these 30 per cent from the rest who do not get IBS, and our preliminary results suggest that psychological factors may make some people particularly susceptible to IBS. It seems that we cannot escape the notion of the mind gut/link even for the IBS that is induced by an attack of gastroenteritis.

Nevertheless, despite the possible psychological link, some of these patients respond very well to anti-inflammatory drugs similar to those used to treat asthma or ulcerative colitis. I have a few patients in whom the condition has been controlled by the drugs Ketotifen or Asacol for several years now. Every time I try to take them off the medication, or even replace it with an identical placebo, the symptoms come back with a vengeance; but they go away when I recommence the treatment.

Food Allergy and Food Intolerance

The popularity of food allergy as a cause of IBS has waxed and waned according to the fashions of time and society. The occasional patient with IBS may indeed have a true food allergy, but I can only think of two such patients in over twenty years' experience of trying to help people with IBS. In both, the ingestion of one particular food constituent, shellfish and nuts respectively in these particular cases, caused the most extreme symptoms of vomiting and diarrhoea and general malaise.

Food intolerance is much more common, to the extent that perhaps everybody with IBS has this to a lesser or greater extent. Food is an extremely important trigger for IBS. It is as if the gut has become sensitive to anything that goes into it or comes out of it. We all know that when we have been out in the sun and our skin has become burnt and sensitive, putting on a shirt will be quite painful. In the same way, if your gut has become sensitive eating food will cause pain and perhaps make the gut try to reject the offending substance by diarrhoea and vomiting, or suppressed forms of these symptoms like a more frequent desire to defecate and indigestion.

Of course, some foods are worse than others. That is not surprising, because we all know that certain foods – spices, fats, onions perhaps, bran or beans – can upset the most tolerant guts. So, if you have guts that are particularly sensitive, such foods are likely to cause excruciating symptoms and are best avoided. It is important to understand, however, that it is not so much the foods that are at fault, more a question of how sensitive the gut is to food in general, and this may vary. Just because that spaghetti bolognaise caused you to go to bed with stomach upset that night your mother came round to dinner, you don't necessarily have to avoid bolognaise sauce forever. It is easy to fall into the pattern of avoiding so many different foods that you could be at serious risk of malnutrition.

This sometimes leads me to question why eating, normally an activity that engenders happiness, comfort and friendship, can become so strongly associated with so much fear and distress. Is this related to a disease of the gut, or is it the result of psychological conditioning by painful associations with food or its provider?

IBS – a Gut Reaction

Mandy's story

'I am just terrified of food,' sobbed Mandy; 'I just had a piece of toast last night and it seemed to stick in my stomach, just there, and it causes the most awful wind.' She made some popping noises with her mouth, finishing off with an impressive belch.

Mandy's symptoms had commenced when she was pregnant with her little girl, Lindy, but got much worse after she was born. Mandy had hardly eaten anything for six weeks and was now just six stone in weight. Mandy had never felt wanted as a child. She didn't know her father and her mother had struggled to bring up three of them on her income from the factory. With Michael out of work, Mandy just didn't know how she would cope with Lindy and Ryan.

In a recent IBS meeting, we asked patients to draw a circle on a sheet of paper and write inside the circle all of the things that made them feel secure and outside the circle all the things that made them feel insecure. They all put 'mother' and 'food' outside the circle. Hardly a scientific study, I acknowledge; nevertheless guilt, anxiety, fear, even terror of eating seems to be an important feature of IBS for so many patients. No, I am not blaming Mum for IBS; not entirely, that is – it's much more complicated that that; but perhaps these observations help us to view IBS from a slightly different perspective. Perhaps we (as doctors) have contributed to the current confusion over IBS by attempting to medicalize it, and treat it with diet, drugs and surgery. To be successful, these approaches must be seen in the context of the personality and life experience of the patient.

This brings us on to the concept of IBS as a reaction of the gut to life events. This would explain quite a lot of things. It would, for example, explain the way in which symptoms can vary from day to day. It would also explain their often symbolic nature. It is amazing how often some of my patients will complain of being unable to 'stomach' the things that are happening to them in their lives when they are suffering nausea or vomiting, whereas other patients may sometimes express a great deal of anger ('getting rid of all that shit!') when they have diarrhoea. The notion of IBS as a gut reaction would also help us to understand why the symptoms tend to be intermittent and episodic, why patients can have good days and bad days, and how frequently recurrence of symptoms is related to life events or emotional upsets, tension, anxiety, depression, anger and so on. The gut can appear to be such a sensitive barometer to what is going on in life that at times it seems as if there is a direct link between the gut and the emotional part of the brain.

I do not think I necessarily see an unusual group of patients with the Irritable Bowel Syndrome; but, having given myself time to listen to them and find out about their lives, I am surprised and saddened by the burden of difficulty, tension and tragedy that many of them seem to have to shoulder and by how many have had to cope with the most awful experiences even from the early stages of childhood. Would I hear the same catalogue of tragedy if I interviewed a random sample of people living in Sheffield? Has life for everybody really become like a script from *Eastenders*? I find that difficult to believe. Several studies have shown that patients with IBS have more anxiety and more depression, and have experienced more severe life events than patients with organic gastrointestinal disease or healthy people.

I do not mean to imply by this that IBS is totally a psychological disease. I think it is a condition that lies between the mind and the gut, and may be initiated by mental or gastrointestinal upset but always involves both. When we bear in mind the strong links between the gut and the emotional side of the brain, it is likely that psychological factors will have a greater effect on a gut that has already been sensitized by disease. After all, we are very familiar with the nausea that can accompany anxiety, the diarrhoea that can accompany apprehension, the choking and difficulty we may have in swallowing when we are upset, the constipation associated with depression. These are aspects of everyday life; they just seem to be much worse in people with Irritable Bowel Syndrome.

If the most useful way of regarding IBS is as a gut reaction, then there seem to be two treatment strategies. The first is to use specific drugs to treat the individual symptoms; the second is to use psychotherapeutic methods to deal with the gut/mind complex. Psychotherapeutic methods are tackled in chapters 4 and 5 of this book, so here I will confine myself to a consideration of symptomatic treatment.

Symptomatic Treatment

'The pains I call the gripes catch me under the ribs on the right side and cause me to double up and take my breath away. Colofac helps these but has no effect on the soreness or what I call wind pains.'

'The only thing I can do when the pain is bad is to lie curled up in bed with a hot water bottle against my tummy.'

There is no therapeutic trial that has ever convincingly demonstrated the efficacy of any drug in IBS.

Abdominal Pain

Anti-spasmodics are currently the mainstay of treatment of Irritable Bowel Syndrome. The pain of IBS is thought to be related to spasm of the colonic muscle and anti-spasmodics, as the name suggests, reduce the strength of gut contraction. There are several anti-spasmodics available; they vary in their potency and side effects. Those that are most commonly prescribed include Colofac (mebeverin), Spasmanol (alverine citrate) and Buscopan (hyoscine butylbromide). Some, in particular Buscopan, may have side effects such as a dry mouth, a little blurring of vision or difficulty in passing urine. Unfortunately, although they may take the edge off the pain, many patients do not seem to find them helpful. In recent years, products containing peppermint oil (Colpermin or Mintec) have become available for treating IBS. Some patients like these, but in general they do not seem to be particularly effective, although patients who suffer with flatuence may notice that their anal expulsions smell more sweetly of peppermint.

More general painkillers such as Panadol, codeine and Distalgesic and particularly the stronger ones such as morphine and Temgesic, have a constipating action. Constipation makes patients with IBS very uncomfortable; so taking these analgesics may create a particularly vicious cycle of pain and constipation. Chronic pain is exhausting; it saps confidence and self-esteem and creates depression. Painkillers may help, but are best kept for emergencies only. Pain is a lot worse if you are anxious or tense. Taking time to relax and rest, maybe with a hot water bottle held close to the abdomen, can help. Relaxation and self-hypnosis tapes can be especially useful. Acupuncture and skin stimulation with TENS machines can also help some people.

Diarrhoea

Diarrhoea can be treated with substances like loperamide (Imodium), Lomotil or codeine phosphate. These are quite powerful and can arrest the flow of the most severe diarrhoea. Unfortunately, patients with bad IBS often find that treatment of their diarrhoea with these agents is complicated by a very marked increase in abdominal pain, as if the diarrhoea had been responsible in some way for relieving the tension within the bowel. Too many anti-diarrhoeal tablets can lead to constipation, and alterating between diarrhoea and constipation is even less pleasant than having either symptom alone.

The most commonly taken drug for diarrhoea is Imodium (loperamide), which can also be bought over the counter as Arrete. Imodium slows down the passage of waste through the system, increases absorption of water and can be very useful if you suffer from urgency or faecal incontinence. Imodium acts on the gut alone and is not absorbed into the system, so side effects are unlikely. Lomotil and (particularly) codeine phosphate are absorbed and can cause side effects of drowsiness or dizziness, and even dependency. All of these drugs are members of the opiate family, like morphine, and those that are absorbed into the system are potentially addictive, though not nearly to the same extent as morphine or heroin.

Questran, as indicated above, can be quite useful in treating frequent watery diarrhoea but is poorly tolerated by most patients with IBS. Bulking agents such as Fybogel, Regulan or Celevac have been advocated for use in diarrhoea as well as constipation on the grounds that they mop up excess fluid. My impression, however, is that they often tend to make the diarrhoea of IBS worse rather then better.

Constipation

The constipation of IBS can usually be treated quite simply with extra fibre in the diet from cereals, fruit and vegetables, or by taking bulking agents. Regulan, Metamucil, Fybogel and Isogel are the most commonly taken; whichever is used, it is important to take it with plenty of water. Linseeds, which can be bought from health food shops, have the same effect. Tolerance to these various substances seems to vary. For some reason I do not understand, my patients seem to prefer Regulan to Fybogel.

Bulking agents ease the passage of waste matter through the system by retaining water and thus making the stools softer and easier to expel. Unfortunately, as explained above, they produce gas, causing distension and may make symptoms of abdominal pain, bloating, flatuence and diarrhoea much worse. Not surprisingly, the sensitive guts of IBS sufferers do not tolerate 'roughage' and gaseous distension very well. It is necessary to experiment with the dose of these agents to obtain the optimum benefit.

Irritant laxatives, such as Sennokot, Dulcolax and Normacol Plus, act by stimulating strong propulsive contractions in the colon. They may have to be given to get the really stubborn gut going, but they can produce the most excruciating spasms in the sensitive colons of patients with IBS. It is best to avoid them if at all possible. Often antispasmodics have to be taken to relieve the discomfort of the laxatives.

Duphalac (Lactulose) is an osmotic laxative: it encourages the secretion of fluid into the bowel and flushes out the obstruction. In the colon, it is fermented to produce a lot of gas. Patients with IBS do not tolerate lactulose very well. The sweet syrup often produces feelings of nausea, and the gas production causes cramping, flatuence and bloating.

The guts of people with IBS are often as sensitive to medications as they are to foods. Even a mild laxative agent such as lactulose or a bulk filler may tip them over into the most painful wind and diarrhoea. It is not just a mechnical problem of getting the dose right; it seems as if the sensitive and turbulent guts of IBS are not going to respond to a simple exercise in hydraulics.

Gassy Symptoms

These are often difficult to treat. There is no definitive treatment for bloating, distension and flatulence, although I often advise patients to cut down on gas-forming foods such as fruit, beans and other pulses, vegetables and cereal fibre (all the stuff that nutritionists have been telling us for twenty years is good!), and avoid bulk-forming laxatives such as Regulan. As explained above, some of the gassiest people in the world are intolerant of milk sugar or lactose: it is always important to enquire about the intake of milk or milk products since a reduction can alleviate this symptom quite remarkably. Treatments for gas are more a matter of avoiding certain foods than taking medicines to absorb gases. Charcoal biscuits and simethicone are prescribed for excessive gas, though I have yet to meet anybody who has said these treatments are effective. But help may be on the way. Beano – no, not the comic – contains the enzyme, alpha-galactosidase, that breaks down vegetable fibre in the small intestine and leads to the absorption of sugars without formation of gas.

> Studies sponsored by the manufacturer, anecdotal reports from scores of people who tried it on their own and personal experience strongly suggest that use of the product, aptly dubbed beano, can greatly reduce the gaseous legacy of many vegetable foods. (*New York Times*)

Beano is not available on prescription and is not to my knowledge marketed in the UK, but if experience in the United States continues to be so positive, it will certainly come here.

Balancing Symptomatic Treatment

Symptomatic treatment is so much a question of balance: fibre improves constipation but makes distension worse, loperamide helps diarrhoea but may worse pain, painkillers help pain but worsen constipation. This causes frustration for both the patient and the doctor. The patient feels that the doctor has really not understood the condition, while the doctor is frustrated by the inability of the conventional medical model, in which he or she has trained, to deal with the large numbers of patients that seem to suffer from gut reactions.

The Placebo Problem

One of the most striking phenomena associated with IBS is its high placebo reactivity. This is the problem that has bedevilled most therapeutic trials in IBS. How can you demonstrate that the new wonder drug, Polodium, is effective against the abdominal pain of Irritable Bowel Syndrome when a 'so-called' inactive placebo relieves pain in up to 60 per cent of sufferers? The wonder drug would have to relieve more than 80 per cent of patients before we could be sure it was effective, and there is no anti-spasmodic or analgesic as good as that. It is said, on not terribly good evidence, that the 'placebo effect' wears off after about three months. That seems to correspond with my own experience.

'You know them tablets, that you gave me last time, doctor? Well, I thought we'd cracked it. I were marvellous the first week, then the pain came back a bit and now I feel just as bad as I did when I first came to see you.'

This is so soul-destroying, not only for the patient but for the doctor as well. What does s/he do? Try another tablet with the almost certain knowledge that the same thing will happen? Is it any wonder that both partners in this therapeutic interaction are frustrated? The most important thing is to avoid the spiral of care that can lead to surgical mutilation, extreme diets and colonic lavage. But that seems very negative and defensive. Is there a more positive approach?

Placebo responsiveness is linked to the power of suggestion, so perhaps it is possible to harness this suggestion to produce more prolonged relief. This is why hypnotherapy is such a powerful and useful method of managing IBS (see chapter 5). It works, not by punitive dieting, invasive testing, traumatic surgery or poisonous drugs, but by quelling fear, establishing confidence and providing support. Whoever said that medicines had to be nasty anyway? Symptoms do not have to be tortured into submission. Their fear and anger can be quelled with kindness.

Treating the Mind/Gut Axis

To date, the most effective means of managing Irritable Bowel Syndrome have been psychotherapeutic techniques. In patients with mild forms of irritable bowel that come on in discrete attacks associated with life events, treatment may simply take the form of empathy, insight and advice; but to undertake this effectively, doctors and other health workers need time to establish effective rapport with the patient, and unfortunately time is one commodity that is in very short supply in our current National Health Service. Other patients may be treated with tranquillizers or anti-depressants. Sleep disturbance is very common in patients with IBS, and many patients take sleeping tablets. Patients with particularly disturbing or chronic symptoms may benefit from more intensive forms of psychotherapy. These include bowel-directed hypnotherapy (see chapter 5) exploratory dynamic psychotherapy and cognitive–behavioural therapy (see chapter 4). The cost-effectiveness of these forms of therapy may be enhanced if they are carried out with groups of patients rather than on an individual basis.

Tranquillizers and Anti-Depressants

Tranquillizers are often prescribed for sufferers of IBS, and they can be helpful. Librium and Valium are the most familiar – the 'mother's little helpers' of the popular song. These drugs have come in for a good deal of adverse publicity in recent years, and rightly so. Some experts say that tranquillizers don't help with the stress that is often associated with IBS because they often reduce the capacity to deal with problems. They also induce dependence, and when somebody successfully stops taking them the withdrawal symptoms can be extremely troublesome. They should therefore only be prescribed in short-term treatments. Side effects include drowsiness, confusion, unsteadiness, visual disturbances, alterations in sex drive and retention of urine. More benefit is obtained by relaxation or stress-management techniques and the opportunity to discuss problems and stresses with a trained counsellor. Many areas provide adult education classes in stress management and relaxation.

Depression is very commonly associated with IBS, and anti-depressant medication can be very useful, especially when combined with practical help to sort out problems and deal with stresses. Anti-depressant medicines are particularly useful in patients with severe chronic pain, as they seem to have a rather specific effect on pain perception. Anti-depressant drugs differ in their strength and side effects, but they do not seem to be blighted by the same degree of dependency and withdrawal problems as tranquillizers. The drugs commonly prescribed to IBS patients include dothiepin (Prothiaden), tofranil (Imipramine) and tryptizol (Amitryptiline). They all cause side effects of dry mouth, constipation, blurred vision, drowsiness, dizziness, weight change and loss of sex drive. Bolvidon is a new type of drug with fewer side effects, though drowsiness can still be a problem.

Hope for the Future

Drugs for the Mind/Gut

Our knowledge about the way the mind and brain may influence the gut is increasing very rapidly, and it is possible that in the future there may be drugs that act on the brain to calm down the irritable gut. In fact, some recent research has shown that a substance called 'leuprolide', which acts on the hypothalamus at the base of the brain to influence the release of sex steroids, can calm down gut reactions in women. This discovery may help to explain why Irritable Bowel Syndrome and other gut reactions appear to be more common in women than they are in men. Other substances currently being investigated act on the gut to reduce sensitivity, rather like anaesthetics. Ondansetron is one of these substances, but is currently only available for the treatment of vomiting induced by chemotherapy; fedotizine is another. By reducing gut feelings these agents may also reduce gut reactions, including emotional consequences.

The link between the gut and emotions goes both ways: emotional upsets appear to be able to make the gut more sensitive and reactive, and gut sensations can influence our emotions, pain inducing anxiety and satiety being associated with a feeling of sleepiness and calm. I feel that there will be some exciting developments in our understanding of the relationship between the brain and the gut in the near future.

'Breaking the Mould'

The major difficulty in managing Irritable Bowel Syndrome is the sheer number of patients with the condition. It has been estimated that about 50 per cent of referrals to gastroenterologists suffer from 'gut reactions' such as IBS, non-specific indigestion, chronic abdominal pain, chronic constipation, chronic diarrhoea and so on. Bearing in mind how difficult it is to treat these conditions by a medical model, this is an enormous burden on the health services. No wonder doctors and patients get frustrated. Is there another way of dealing with the problem? I think there is, namely, to work with groups to educate and provide insights into the management of IBS.

There is no standard way of conducting group management of IBS. The model we have developed in our department at Sheffield incorporates between eight and ten evening meetings, each lasting about two to two and a half hours. The first two meetings are educational and use visual aids as well as discussion to explore areas such as: What is IBS? When should you be worried that this is not IBS and something that needs further investigation? The role of diet in IBS; the role of stress; medical management; stress management and relaxation. These educational sessions are aimed at enabling patients to manage the disease themselves. In the remaining sessions the patients are encouraged to think about their symptoms in relation to their life experiences. We have used a number of devices to encourage this. The circle of security, described above in relation to 'mother' and 'food', is one. In another exercise, patients draw an outline of themselves and within each part of the body put a diagrammatic representation of what that part feels like. These simple techniques often generate discussion of the symbolic significance of the symptoms in relation to previous life events. At the end of each group session, there is a period of relaxation; it is possible that simple hypnotic techniques could be used to enhance this.

These groups need not be run by consultants or medical experts in IBS; they could be run by members of the health team who have had some training in counselling and group skills. After a time they could be facilitated by patients who have been members of previous groups. The idea is that the groups would be seeded by the team and would then propagate throughout the region. This is an area where health workers and patient self-help groups could work together very successfully. Our initial results are encouraging.

Conclusion

I feel that the way in which diseases like Irritable Bowel Syndrome are regarded by patients and doctors alike is undergoing a quiet revolution. There is a growing realization that the conventional and traditional management of Irritable Bowel Syndrome according to a medical model does not really work. Doctors, therapists and other health workers need to work with patient self-help groups to bring about a change in management of the condition. Self-help groups, like the IBS Network, are in the vanguard of this movement, and can help to bring about this change. It is very important, however, that they work in collaboration with health workers.

The medical model may be criticized for being patriarchal and closed-minded, but self-help without training and guidance can lead to confusion. To my mind, we are more certain now of what IBS is and how to manage it than we have ever been. Over the last thirty years IBS has been regarded as a disease of fibre deficiency, a motility disorder and a disturbance of gastrointestinal sensitivity; but now it is being increasingly regarded as a psychosomatic condition: either the gastrointestinal expression of psychic conflict, in which mental torment is focused on the gut because it is intolerable to accept it in the mind, or a gut sensitized by disease to the gut-wrenching influence of psychological factors. In my experience, the former seems more likely, but this is the one that is rejected by many IBS sufferers. Indeed, it would have to be: somebody who has subconsciously converted suppressed traumatic experience into gut symptoms to avoid intense anxiety or depression is likely to resist strenuously any attempt to unmask any psychological mechanism that may lie behind the symptoms. Talking to patients with IBS can be like opening Pandora's Box; the most awful tragedies and problems lie buried in there. Would the same problems exist in representative samples of healthy people or patients with other gastrointestinal disorders such as Crohn's Disease? Is this just what our life is in post-industrial societies? I do not think so. Studies have shown that patients with IBS seem to have experienced more traumatic life events than patients with other gastrointestinal disease or healthy subjects.

The management of IBS can appear to be in a state of confusion because health workers and patients shy away from seeing it for what it is – a disease at the interaction of the mind and the gut. Such conditions have long been regarded as not being 'proper diseases', and patients dismissed with the admonition that they should 'pull themselves together'. It is time that IBS is treated seriously without fear or prejudice. It is not the patient that is the failure; it is the medical model that is inappropriate. Acknowledgement of this must pave the way for more sympathetic and effective treatment.

3

Can You Have Your Cake and Eat It? Dietary Treatment of IBS

Alan Stewart and Maryon Stewart

Irritable Bowel Syndrome is a very common condition which though not life-threatening can have a profound effect on the quality of life. As chapters 1 and 2 have indicated, there are numerous ideas as to its causes: many experts, however, are of the opinion that IBS is commonly influenced by two main external factors: stress, and what we eat. Both these factors have the potential to influence the normal functioning of the muscles in the bowel and thereby influence the symptoms of IBS.

The evidence that IBS or the symptoms of IBS are influenced by what you eat comes essentially from three different types of study: studies that look at the effect of fibre-rich foods on the gut in healthy people and those with IBS; studies of diets that initially exclude a large number of foods and try to determine the influence of individual foods or food groups when they are reintroduced into the diet; and studies that look at the effect of individual foods on gut function, either in the normal population or in those with a bowel problem (but not always IBS). These rather mixed sources of information do now allow us to have some idea of the role that diet can play in IBS.

An important and sometimes confusing issue is that of food intolerance and food allergy. There is much controversy as to how common genuine adverse reactions to food are. The word 'allergy' is reserved for those reactions that involve the person's immune system, such as those that occur in asthma, eczema and nettle-rash, and sometimes with bowel-related problems. True food allergy can be immediate, as in reactions to peanuts causing lip swelling and asthma, or delayed, taking perhaps several days before there is a discernible reaction to cow's milk protein or wheat. This can sometimes be the case in IBS. More common, though, are food 'intolerances', where eating or drinking the item in question can result in bowel or other symptoms. The immune system is not involved and the adverse reaction involves a chemical effect of the food, as for example when the caffeine in tea and coffee aggravates anxiety, causes palpitations or influences some bowel symptoms. Cow's milk sugar, lactose, is not digested by some and consequently stimulates diarrhoea because it chemically attracts water into the gut. This is an example of an inability to tolerate a certain chemical component of a food. Intolerances can occur to a number of dietary items and these may be factors in an unknown proportion of those with IBS.

In an ideal world there would be some simple test that would provide us with a quick and accurate assessment of food allergies and intolerances. This is not the case, nor is it likely to be so in the near future. Very often an assessment of these problems is first made by the person following a few-foods diet or exclusion diet for two or three weeks. Such diets are typically composed of some meats, a few fruits and vegetables, rice instead of wheat and bread, soya milk instead of cow's, and water instead of tea and coffee. If benefit is obtained after a short while the careful introduction of specific excluded foods at three- to four-day intervals may allow the sufferer to identify those dietary elements that aggravate their symptoms. At times certain food allergies can be assessed by use of blood and skin tests, but these are not frequently undertaken.

It would seem from published research that this type of approach has achieved significant success in treating IBS. Such diets are best followed under the supervision of an experienced doctor or dietetic adviser, though more simple versions may not always require this. They should not be undertaken by those who are underweight, children, pregnant or breastfeeding women, the elderly, those with a history of eating disorders or serious depression, diabetics or anyone with any serious current illness, without medical assessment and guidance. Additionally, those who have lost weight, have been eating poorly, are already on a restricted diet or have symptoms suggestive of nutritional deficiencies such as fatigue, depression, recurrent mouth ulcers, cracking of the lips or muscle pains may well need nutritional supplements. The need for this should be assessed before an exclusion diet is undertaken and medical involvement is again necessary.

To make sense of the use of dietary manipulation in treating IBS we need to look at the symptoms of irritable bowel and how they are caused. However, before leaving the topic of allergy and intolerance we must point out an important guiding principle. There is an enormous amount of individual variation in reactions to foods. This means that two people with IBS, even two who have the same symptoms, may respond to quite different dietary measures. One may respond to one kind of dietary change and the other may respond to a different diet, or may not benefit at all from dietary manipulation but may gain from some other type of approach. It is individual assessment that seems to produce the best results.

Diet and the Symptoms of IBS

By understanding how the symptoms of IBS can be caused we can gain some insight as to how our diet, and in particular how some particular foods and beverages may cause or contribute to their production.

The symptoms of IBS have been described in chapter 1 of this book. To summarize, the common features of the condition are abdominal pain; a change in frequency of bowel movement, either 'diarrhoea' (more than three stools per day) or 'constipation' (fewer than three stools per week); a change in stool consistency; a change in how it feels to pass stools; passage of mucus in stools; slime in the stool; and abominal bloating (usually with wind).

Looking at these one by one, we can suggest explanations likely.

Pain

The pain felt in IBS can be anything from a mild ache to a severe cramp and can be felt almost anywhere in the abdomen or can be felt as low back or pelvic pain. This pain seems to be mainly due to an excessive build-up in pressure in the gut when the muscles of the gut fail to contract in a smooth and regular fashion. A wave of contraction passing down the gut reaches a segment which is already in spasm. There is then a substantial rise in pressure inside the gut as the 'unstoppable force' meets the 'immovable object'. A high level of pressure inside the gut itself tenses the wall and this causes pain.

This explanation as to the cause of the pain has been confirmed by experiments in which volunteers have swallowed a fine tube with a balloon on the end. When this is inflated, it presses on the walls of the intestine and causes pain. Often a point somewhere in the small bowel can be found where inflation of the balloon exactly reproduces the pain that that person experiences as part of his or her IBS. So pain can be due to a rise in pressure inside the gut.

In those with true food allergy there can be a release of chemicals from the wall of the bowel that produce inflammation. These chemicals are the same as those that are produced in arthritis and other situations where the tissues are irritated and trying to heal. They could certainly contribute to or aggravate the pain of IBS.

Diarrhoea

The term diarrhoea is used to describe excessively frequent or loose bowel movements. 'Frequent' means more than three stools per day, and 'loose' means anything from the consistency of soft putty to watery. Diarrhoea mainly comes about because food has moved too quickly through the gut so that there has not been time for the water in the bowel to be absorbed. Though you might think that diarrhoea would often be accompanied by an increase in the activity of the muscles of the gut, this does not appear always to be the case: the gut muscles may be *less* active as food passes through unimpeded by gut contractions.

Diarrhoea can certainly be due to dietary factors, including:

- true food allergy, where there is a reaction to a food involving the immune system as in reaction to wheat protein or cow's milk protein;
- food intolerance, where the food may irritate the gut without involving the immune system, perhaps because of an inability to digest and absorb the food or part of it, as in lactose (cow's milk sugar) intolerance or fruit sugar intolerance;
- a direct chemical or drug-like effect on the gut, as with tea or coffee.

Diarrhoea, if prolonged, could lead to a lack of some nutrients, but this rarely occurs in IBS.

Constipation

Constipation is defined as infrequent passage of stools, usually three times a week or fewer, but may also refer to difficult or incomplete evacuation of the bowels. It is a common problem for those living in industrialized countries. Modern lifestyles, with a relatively poor intake of fibre-rich foods and a low level of physical activity, are thought by many to be important in the development of constipation, with or without the other features of IBS.

Constipation is due not to lack of muscle activity but rather to the wrong kind. There would appear to be a lack of regular coordinated waves of relaxation and contraction passing along the gut. Instead, there may be areas of heightened activity resulting in spasm, which may then impede the regular gut action. Furthermore, the muscles at the lower end of the bowel that you use to help push when you open your bowels may not be very strong, or conversely may be in spasm too. So constipation in IBS may signify disturbance in muscle function.

Constipation can result from a variety of dietary factors, including:

- a lack of fibre-rich foods, the bulk of which in the large bowel helps to stimulate normal waves of muscle activity;
- food allergy, when irritation of the bowel might induce localized spasm that interferes with normal bowel muscle activity;
- possibly a lack of other factors in our diet, such as foods that are natural laxatives and vegetables that are rich not only in fibre but also in magnesium, a traditional and simple laxative.

There is another aspect to severe constipation, especially in women, that deserves consideration. A number of studies have revealed that this symptom can be associated with other health problems, including breast lumps and precancerous changes in breast tissue; hormonal abnormalities (e.g. low oestrogen level); more painful and irregular periods; a greater chance of hysterectomy or operation for a cyst on the ovary; pain on intercourse and difficulty achieving orgasm; infertility; hesitancy in starting to pass water; cold hands and a tendency to faint. Curiously, the group of women who suffer with these problems do not tend to eat less fibre than other women. These diverse health problems can be explained by the important part that the bowel plays in the metabolism (breaking down) of the female sex hormone, oestrogen. Many of the women who suffer from these conditions appear to have poorly coordinated and excessive contraction of the muscles around the lower end of the bowel, vagina and bladder.

Wind and Bloating

Excessive wind and abdominal bloating are common symptons that often go together. By wind is meant flatus, or gas passed through the back passage. Burping or, to give it its medical term, eructation, can also occur as part of IBS and is usually due to the swallowing of air.

Flatus comes from the breakdown of food residues in the colon and also from the residue of mucus or digestive slime and juices that our own intestines produce. Gases are produced by the billions of mainly friendly bacteria that inhabit our large colon. They are found only in very small amounts in the small bowel where the majority of digestion and absorption of nutrients takes place. They first appear in any quantity in the caecum, which is the first part of the large bowel. Here the bacteria are waiting to see what will turn up in the form of left-overs from the meal that you have eaten several hours before. This normally constitutes about 5–10 per cent of our intake of fat, protein and carbohydrate as well as all of the fibre. The bacteria break down the fibre and food residues, releasing a small amount of energy and some acids, and producing gases that our own cells are, for the most part, incapable of producing. These include hydrogen, methane and some carbon dioxide, all of which have no smell. In some people and under certain circumstances 'bad-eggs' gas, hydrogen sulphide, is produced – an event with which some of us are doubtless familiar. Also in the colon a large amount of water and a small amount of some minerals are slowly absorbed.

There is quite a lot of activity in the normal colon, then. We all have some wind; the degree and type depend on:

- the type of food eaten, especially whether fibre-rich foods are included;
- how well the food is digested in the small bowel;
- how quickly food and food residues pass through the small bowel to reach the colon;
- the type of bacteria present in the colon;

- whether you have eaten foods to which you are allergic or intolerant.

The Fibre Question

Until the late 1970s IBS was commonly considered to be best treated by a diet *low* in 'roughage' (vegetable fibre). Then came the observations of Dr Painter, a British naval surgeon who noticed the association between a high fibre intake and an absence of many of the diseases of civilization, of which IBS was one. Perhaps, it began to be thought, a lack of fibre might be the cause of irritable bowel? In recent years a number of experts and expert committees have recommended that the British population as a whole should increase its fibre intake by about 40 per cent. This would mean eating on average about 40 per cent more fruit, vegetables and cereals (bread and other foods containing wheat, oat, barley, rye and sweet corn/maize).

Several studies have also shown that the larger the intake of dietary fibre, the larger is the resultant output of stool; and the larger the output of stool, the quicker is the passage of food from one end of the body to the other, known as the 'gut transit time'. However, not everyone obeys these simple rules. Girls' bowels move more slowly than boys', and some girls have very slow bowels despite a reasonable fibre intake. So, though increasing fibre intake always increases the weight of the stool, the effect of this can be quite variable; and, as you may already know, fibre is not always the answer to constipation and IBS.

Individual Foods/Drinks and IBS

Now we can look at how particular foods might be contributing to some of your IBS symptoms. In the sections that follow we will give you enough information to make what is essentially an informed guess about different foods and beverages. Remember that the biggest unknown factor in all of this is your particular, individual response to a particular food. So the acid test is: how does it effect *you* when you eat it?

Table 1   A summary of the possible influence of individual foods on the symptoms of IBS

| | Symptom | | |
Food/Beverage	Constipation	Diarrhoea	Wind
Cow's Milk	Rarely	Due to lactose intolerance	As for diarrhoea
Wheat, especially wholewheat and wheat bran	Surprisingly common	Certainly	With diarrhoea or constipation
Oats, barley and rye	As for wheat but usually less marked		
Sweet corn (maize)	–	Especially if not well chewed	As for diarrhoea
Tea	Definitely	–	–
Coffee	–	Definitely	Possibly
Alcohol	Unlikely	Definitely	Possible 'bad eggs'
Yeast-rich foods	Uncertain	Possible	–
Fruits generally	Unlikely	Too much fruit sugar (fructose)	As for diarrhoea
Citrus fruits	Unlikely	Possible	–
Honey	Unlikely	If you ate a lot	–
Sugar (sucrose)	–	Very rarely	–
Sorbitol (sweetener)	–	If you eat too much	–
Beans	Unlikely	Especially if not cooked thoroughly	Very possible
Onions	–	Possible	Possible 'bad eggs'
Green vegetables	Unlikely	Possible	Quite possible
Fatty foods	Unlikely	Possible if rapid gut transit	As for diarrhoea
Eggs	According to folk lore	Possible but rare?	Quite possible
Anything else	Possible	Possible	Possible

Note: A dash indicates no known effect.

Milk

Milk can cause bowel problems, and in particular diarrhoea, in one of two ways. Some people, especially children and infants, may react to the protein in milk and this can cause abdominal pain (or colic in an infant), and sometimes diarrhoea. Other signs of allergy may be eczema, asthma or a blocked or runny nose.

Sometimes there can be a problem with milk sugar (lactose). If this cannot be digested then the sugar passes into the small bowel and colon, where it acts as a potent laxative. The severely affected sufferer is frequently troubled with diarrhoea, often with wind, within a hour of consuming milk or soft cheese. Hard cheese or small amounts of milk may be tolerated. This type of food intolerance is quite common in those of east European, Middle Eastern or Asian origin, and in others following an episode of acute gastroenteritis. Drinking skimmed or semi-skimmed milk makes no difference to either cow's milk protein or lactose intolerance as it is only the fat content that is reduced in these milks, not the protein or sugar content.

Constipation seems to be less of a problem but is certainly possible in those with cow's milk protein intolerance.

Wheat and other grains

It now seems that wheat, together with the other grains, oats, barley and rye, which all contain a protein called gluten, is one of the foods that most aggravates the symptoms of IBS. This has been found in studies of food intolerance where an exclusion diet has been used, but has also been recorded as a cause of diarrhoea, especially in women. This situation is similar to, but distinct from, coeliac disease, in which gluten sensitivity is severe, resulting in damage to the lining of the intestine.

Together with diarrhoea there is often weight loss, anaemia and nutritional deficiencies; constipation can also be a problem, or indeed there may be a combination of the two. Other studies have shown that there is a slowing in the rate at which the stomach empties when whole wheat is eaten, while the high fibre content of whole wheat and wheat bran may speed passage through the colon (large bowel).

Although the first study of the use of wheat bran in treating IBS showed an improvement for most, it was not good for all: some in particular noticed an increase in pain. Subsequently other doctors have revealed a very mixed picture, with extra wheat bran likely to worsen abdominal bloating and wind but to ease constipation. Its only definite use is against simple constipation, but even here it may not suit everyone.

The fibre from fruit and vegetables is just as effective as grain fibre, comes with a good amount and variety of vitamins and minerals, and seems less likely to aggravate IBS symptoms in the majority of patients.

Finally, if you are very sensitive to these grains you may also need to be wary of 'modified starch', shown on the ingredients list of many prepared foods, which may be made from wheat and still cause problems in the very sensitive.

Sweet corn

Maize or sweet corn can also cause problems. It may be tolerated by those who cannot take wheat, oat barley and rye as it does not contain gluten. However, some people do not get on well with it. It is hard to digest unless it is chewed well; indeed, a simple way of working out how long it takes for food to get from one end to the other is to eat sweet corn and not chew it – but watch out for the wind. Cornflakes are made from maize and are often a safe alternative for those who cannot take wheat or oats, but some will still have problems.

Tea

Our favourite beverage does not escape without comment. A study by Scandinavian doctors showed that about half of a group of normal subjects experienced a change in the rate at which food moved through the gut when they replaced their intake of water with tea. For the other half there was no difference. No wonder constipation is described as 'the English disease'. It is likely that if you are regular tea drinker and suffer from constipation as part of your IBS, cutting down on your tea intake and eating a high-fibre diet will be of some benefit. Remember to reduce your tea consumption gradually over a week or two, though, otherwise a caffeine withdrawal headache may well result.

Coffee

This extremely popular beverage is also an excellent bowel stimulant. Both ordinary and decaffeinated coffee have effects on the gut, one of which is to stimulate a wave of contraction along the bowel. Many people use a cup of coffee as a way of helping them to go to the toilet. For some, however, it can actually be a cause of diarrhoea: so if you have diarrhoea and you drink coffee, you should cut down or stop completely – even decaffeinated coffee can affect the gut.

Hot drinks in general can also stimulate a wave of contraction through the bowel, so again it may be necessary to limit the number of such drinks that you have.

Alcohol

Alcohol too can sometimes cause diarrhoea, though this is usually likely to happen only in those who drink very heavily. The safe limit for men is three units per day and for women it is two. Intakes higher than this are associated with a number of health problems from liver disease to an increased risk of cancer. Beer and cheaper wines contain quite a lot of the preservative sulphite which can contribute to the bad-eggs smell in those who are windy. So be warned.

Yeast

Sometimes certain alcoholic beverages may aggravate IBS because of a sensitivity to yeast. This is posible with beer, especially yeasty tasting real ales, and men are more likely to be so troubled than women. You may also find that other yeast-rich foods such as yeast extract, savoury snacks, packet soups and gravies as well as bread can also aggravate the symptoms of IBS.

Fruit and honey

Though you might think that these foods are easy to digest, they may not suit everyone. Fruit, some vegetables and honey are all rich in fructose or fruit sugar, which is not absorbed into the body as quickly as some other sugars. Any remaining in the gut can act as a laxative. Many of us may have experienced problems of bloating, wind and diarrhoea after eating a lot of fruit, especially grapes, dates or other very sweet fruits. The same could happen with a lot of honey. The effect might be more noticeable if several pieces of fruit are eaten on an empty stomach.

About the only fruit consistently to cause problems seems to be oranges, and sometimes grapefruit and lemons. Why this is so is not clear. Certainly all other fruits can occasionally cause a disturbance in bowel function in some sensitive people. Stewing fruit can make it easier to digest, and this may be especially important for older folk.

Sugar

Table sugar (sucrose) only very rarely causes problems. Diarrhoea can result in the few people who have difficulty digesting and absorbing it.

Artificial sweeteners

One artificial sweetener, sorbitol, which is used in some sugar-free chewing gums and sweets (especially mints) can, if consumed excessively, cause diarrhoea. Sorbitol is an 'artificial sugar' which tastes sweet but cannot be digested. It therefore passes through the small bowel intact, moving on to the large bowel where it can attract water in the same way that some mineral laxatives do. So eating too many low-calorie mints can be a cause of diarrhoea.

Beans, onions and green vegetables

All of these foods have a reputation for causing wind. Alas, it is deserved, because they can for some susceptible individuals be hard to digest, and the remaining portion then serves as a food source for the gas-producing bacteria that are lurking in your large bowel. The following foods are all relatively likely to produce wind: vegetables of the Brassica family (cabbage, cauliflower, broccoli, and brussel sprouts); Jerusalem artichokes; onions and other members of this family such as leeks and garlic.

These foods seem more likely to cause wind if they are not well cooked and are eaten in large amounts. Men may be more susceptible to the effect than women because of their faster rate of gut transport.

Fatty foods

Too much fatty food can, if the digestion is poor, lead to diarrhoea. This is not normally a problem in those with IBS. However, any cause of diarrhoea that results in more than three stools a day can be associated with a small loss of nutrients in the stool, and, a high intake of fatty foods could aggravate this. So take care, especially if your diarrhoea is worse a few hours after eating a large or rich meal.

Conversely, fat in more modest quanitites actually slows down the rate at which the stomach empties and food moves along the small bowel. Nature knows that fat in a meal takes time to digest, and so the gut is sensitive to its presence. Certain fats seem particularly good at this 'braking' effect: for example, oleic acid, which is found in olive oil and rapeseed oil. It is thought that too low a fat intake may explain why low-fat diets in children can prolong toddler diarrhoea. If you have diarrhoea, try including small amounts of olive and rapeseed oils in your diet.

Eggs

We know of no good evidence that eggs are 'binding', as some say; nor do we know why they have this reputation for causing constipation. They are, however, prohibited in most exclusion diets, and if you are allergic to them they could as easily cause diarrhoea as constipation.

Anything else
By now you should have the idea that virtually anything you eat could play a part in your IBS. Water seems safe; but there are some who feel that bottled water is better for them. The commonest chemical found in ordinary tap water is chlorine, which is added to kill off bacteria; and it is quickly lost if the water is boiled or left in the open air for an hour or so.

Overall you must trust your own judgement and do not rely too heavily upon the advice of others. Look at the information given here as suggestions, which may lead to an improvement but may not.

Additional Dietary Factors that can Influence the Pattern of IBS Symptoms

Size of meals
Eating a large meal can trigger a reflex contraction of the colon muscles; this explains why you may have felt the need to open your bowels within an hour or so of your main meal of the day. It isn't that meal coming through already, but probably the day before's moving on. Some people with IBS are unduly sensitive in this respect.

Smoking
Smoking a cigarette is known to increase the contraction of the colon muscles in those with IBS. If you smoke, or have been a smoker, you will know that a few puffs can cause a need to open the bowels. For many, a cup of coffee and a cigarette is their way of going to the toilet.

Drugs
Certain drugs and nutritional supplements can cause diarrhoea as a side effect. The obvious clue is if the diarrhoea

started shortly after you started taking the drug/supplement. Stopping it should result in improvement within a few days, though occasionally it may take longer. Anti-arthritic drugs and strong painkillers can irritate the upper or lower parts of the gut and produce severe indigestion or symptoms similar to IBS, usually with diarrhoea. Very large doses of vitamin C and magnesium can also cause diarrhoea, as can yeast tablets, which also cause bloating. Iron preparations and multivitamins with iron can irritate some people's digestion. Antibiotics, especially those of the penicillin family, can cause diarrhoea, almost certainly due to a change in the flora of the colon.

Candida

A build-up in the bowel of the yeast *Candida albicans* can be a factor in IBS. This organism is well known as the cause of thrush, which commonly occurs in the vagina and sometimes in the mouth. It is usually responds to treatment with anti-fungal agents and dietary change. Sometimes an episode of vaginal thrush or infection elsewhere triggers IBS in the first place. The part that this yeast organism may play in IBS has in our opinion been rather overstated in some of the popular press and understated in the mainstream medical journals. It can be found somewhere in the gut of some 20 per cent of the normal population and does not automatically cause bowel symptoms.

Certain factors can encourage a build-up of candida, such as use of antibiotics, treatment with steroids, diabetes, deficiencies of iron and the B vitamins, and possibly a diet high in refined foods and sugar and low in essential nutrients, and this might then lead to bowel and other problems due to this organism. A few people are genuinely allergic to it; this had been reported in cases of urticaria (nettle-rash) and eczema. It would seem that some of those with IBS where diarrhoea and bloating are the main problems may benefit from certain 'anti-candida' measures. These include the use of antibiotic preparations that kill candida, eating a nutritious diet, cutting down on sugar-rich foods and avoiding yeast-rich foods such as bread, alcoholic beverages, vinegar, stock cubes and foods containing yeast extract. Improvement, if it is going to occur, should be evident within a few weeks. It may not be necessary to follow all of these measures indefinitely.

Gut bacteria

Several non-prescription preparations containing friendly *Lactobacillus* bacteria are available. Their effectiveness is very much hit-and-miss and will remain so until scientific appraisal takes place. Similarly, there are some whose food intolerances might be helped by taking enzyme preparations that increase the digestion of wind-producing foods.

Menstruation

Many women notice that in the week before their period their abdomen bloats, they become constipated and they may have some generalized abdominal discomfort. The actual arrival of the period may be associated with diarrhoea. This may be due to the release of chemicals that stimulate the bowel to contract as well as the uterus. Constipation in association with premenstrual syndrome (PMS) may well respond to a change of diet, supplements of multivitamins and quite large doses of the mineral magnesium, which is known to help PMS symptoms, acts as a safe and effective laxative and can be lacking in some 50 per cent of women with PMS.

Evening primrose oil has also been used with some success in IBS, giving modest benefit to a group of women with known food intolerances who despite dietary restriction still experienced symptoms premenstrually and menstrually.

Diet and IBS: Can It Help?

It would seem that there are many factors that can contribute to the symptoms of IBS. Dietary factors look like being the most common – and the most complicated, which element probably explains why there seems to be little agreement about the best way to tackle IBS by diet except for the recommendation to increase fibre intake in those with constipation.

Very often the best way forward for the individual is some trial of dietary change which may or may not be supervised by a doctor or dietitian. The better-informed the therapist and patient are, the greater the likelihood of success. We hope that this chapter, together with the others in this book, will help achieve this.

Finally, it is very likely indeed that future research into the role of diet in IBS will allow better and more specific advice to be given to IBS sufferers; always, of course, remembering that it is the individual who makes the final judgement as to what foods or what factors suit their bowel function.

Three Case Histories

Diarrhoea: Jane

Jane was a 32-year-old veterinary assistant who for five years had experienced episodic and at times quite dramatic diarrhoea. She suspected that wine and dairy products aggravated her problems. However, it was not until she followed a quite strict exclusion diet for three weeks that her residual symptoms disappeared. They quickly returned when some foods were introduced into her diet. Milk resulted in diarrhoea and wind within an hour; cheese, citrus fruits, wine and milk chocolate resulted in diarrhoea and wind that built up over several hours. Being strict with her diet meant that she could stop her anti-diarrhoea drugs, and she also experienced a marked improvement in energy. It was likely that she had a true lactose (milk sugar) intolerance as well as other food intolerances, and it seemed that these had developed gradually over several years.

Constipation: Nicole

Nicole at the age of 30 was fed up with eight years of severe constipation and abdominal bloating. This had followed a bad road accident in which she had fractured her pelvis, after which she did not open her bowels for several weeks. Headaches, malaise and premenstrual problems were also problems for her. There was a surprising degree of improvement when she began a diet that excluded most grains, dairy products, yeast, tea, coffee and several other foods. There was even more improvement when she took supplements of magnesium and multivitamins to correct some mild nutritional deficiences. Over the next seven years she tried on many occasions to reintroduce these foods and always reacted badly to them. Indeed, her sensitivity to wheat became so great that even taking a small amount of biscuit or communion wafer caused mouth soreness within an hour which then developed into mouth ulceration. This pattern was strongly suggestive of a true food allergy. Her avoidance of all dairy products meant that she required a calcium and multivitamin supplement. Interestingly, her level of sensitivity to these foods increased over the years, though it would seem that it is more usual for such reactions to settle down.

Wind: Damien

Damien was a rather oversensitive 56-year-old theatre critic whose abdominal bloating, wind and diarrhoea could easily be put down to his nerves. This seemed likely, as two gastroenterologists had found no serious digestive disorder. However, it seemed worth him trying an exclusion diet, which he dutifully followed but without any significant benefit. The only time he seemed to improve was when he included a lot of milk and eggs in his diet. After several months the only conclusion we could come to was that certain fibrerich foods such as beans and wholemeal bread seemed to make his symptoms worse, though the effect was not dramatic. Further consultations with one of his specialists resulted in some advice to help control the build-up of gas-forming bacteria in the bowel. Taking a specialized preparation of healthy bacteria to reduce the concentration of the undesirable ones seemed to produce lasting and significant benefit after a few months. Damien was then able to tolerate foods that previously had aggravated his symptoms.

Meal Ideas and Recipes
(compiled by Susan Backhouse)

Avoiding those foods which are commonly thought to aggravate IBS symptoms sounds simple enough: you simply cut them out of your diet. However, embarking on a dairy- or gluten-free diet can be more difficult than this suggests, because these foods often make up a major part of our diet. Fortunately, there are many books available dedicated to gluten-free and dairy-free cooking: for suggestions, see the 'Useful Books' section in the Appendix at the end of this book. (This list also contains a book that might be useful for people wishing to go an anti-candida diet, which is out of our scope here.)

If you do want to undertake a restrictive diet, it is advisable to seek the help of a doctor or a nutritionally experienced health practitioner in order to make sure that you don't miss out on essential nutrients. However, there is much that you can do for yourself to ensure that you have a varied and interesting diet.

You can quickly get used to substituting dairy- and gluten-free alternatives for commonly used ingredients. For example:

- instead of cow's milk, use goat's or sheep's milk, soya or nut milk ($\frac{1}{4}$ cup ground nuts with $1\frac{1}{4}$ cup water);
- instead of cheese and yoghurt made with cow's milk, use equivalent made with goat's, sheep's or soya milk;
- instead of butter and margarine, use dairy-free margarine (e.g. Whole Earth's 'Superspread', which does not contain hydrogenated fats) or cold-pressed oil;

- instead of ordinary flours and cereals, use rice, millet, soya (usually mixed with other flours), buckwheat (though this is strong-tasting and needs to be got used to), potato, gram, corn (maize), spelt, sago and tapioca (these last two tend to go 'glutinous' when used in sauces);
- use gluten-free baking powder: many baking powders do contain gluten, but at the time of writing Sainsbury's does not; also try wholefood shops for the gluten-free type.

Remember when you are buying ingredients and prepared foods to check labels carefully: there are often 'hidden' ingredients where you would not expect them. For example, monosodium glutamate contains gluten.

Many other useful ingredients are widely available, though you may have to go to different shops for them, for example:

- tahini (sesame paste) can be bought in Greek food shops, wholefood shops and some supermarkets;
- tofu (soybean curd) can be bought in Chinese food shops and wholefood shops;
- tamari (strong soya sauce that does not, as do many soya sauces, contain wheat) can be bought in oriental food shops and wholefood shops;
- agar-agar (a vegetarian gelling agent) can be bought in wholefood shops.

You can also adapt your established cooking methods to incorporate the alternative ingredients. For example:

- crumbles can be made with ground nuts, either on their own or mixed with brown rice flour, seeds, millet flakes and/or dessicated coconut (though check that this last is gluten-free);
- if you are avoiding milk or eggs, try mixing soya flour with a little water to make a glaze for pastry;
- it is a good idea to combine different types of gluten-free flours for baking – e.g. three-quarters rice flour with one-eighth each of corn flour and buckwheat flour;
- as pastry made with gluten-free flour tends to disintegrate

easily, it helps if you roll it out between sheets of grease-proof paper;
- you can make bread without yeast using an ingredient called 'Arise'.*

The remainder of this chapter gives some meal ideas and recipes for people who want to avoid dairy produce and wheat or gluten. To help you find the recipes to suit you, each heading is marked **DF** (dairy-free) or **GF** (gluten-free), or both, as appropriate. Weights and measures are given in both metric and imperial terms: stick to one system throughout each recipe.

Breakfasts
- Cereals with soya milk or fruit juice (**DF**)
- Toast with dairy-free margarine or nut butter (**DF**)
- Porridge made out of rice flakes, millet flakes, buckwheat flakes. Flavour with cinnamon, cloves and dates or fresh fruit, chopped nuts and seeds (**DF/GF**)
- Rice cakes with mashed bananas, almond or other nut butter and Whole Earth sugar-free fruit spread (**DF/GF**)
- Rice cakes with tahini and Marmite (**DF/GF**)
- Vitality Shake: mix equal measures of milk or soya milk and orange juice; liquidize and add 1 tsp brewer's yeast and 1 tsp molasses; blend until smooth and serve chilled (**DF/GF**)
- Gluten-free Muesli (see recipe below)

Gluten-free Muesli (**DF/GF**)
(from *The Neal's Yard Bakery Wholefood Cookbook* by Rachel Haigh)

> 500 g (1 lb 2 oz) rice flakes
> 500 g (1 lb 2 oz) millet flakes
> 250 g (9 oz) sunflower seeds

* 'Arise' is available from: Cirrus Associates (South West), Little Hintock, Kington Magna, Gillingham, Dorset SP8 5EW.

250 g (9 oz) raisins
250 g (9 oz) sultanas
250 g (9 oz) hazelnuts
250 g (9 oz) dried apricots
90 ml (6 tbsp) desiccated coconut
250 g (9 oz) soya bran (optional, for added fibre)

Combine the ingredients and store in a airtight jar in a cool place. Serve with milk, yoghurt, soya milk or fruit juice; add a little fresh fruit if wished. Eat immediately or leave to soak overnight. Alternatively, cover with your choice of liquid, simmer gently for five minutes and eat warm.
Makes 2.5 kg (4 lb 6 oz).

Starters and Light Lunches or Suppers

Guacamole (**DF/GF**)
(from *The Neal's Yard Bakery Wholefood Cookbook* by Rachel Haigh)

This traditional Mexican dish needs really well-ripened avocados.

3 avocados
1 large tomato, finely chopped
juice and grated rind of 1 lemon
pinch of chilli powder or cayenne pepper
15 ml (1 tbsp) olive oil (optional)
salt and black pepper
black olives to garnish

1. Put the avocado flesh into a mixing bowl and mash with a fork or a potato masher.
2. Add the tomato and the lemon juice and rind.
3. Sprinkle over the chilli and olive oil, if using, and season to taste.
4. Garnish with black olives.

Serves 6.

Hummus (**DF/GF**)
(from *The Neal's Yard Bakery Wholefood Cookbook* by Rachel Haigh)

A blender is essential for this recipe. Make sure the chickpeas are thoroughly cooked before liquidizing. Chickpeas can be soaked for two to three days, which can help to avoid causing flatulence. Change the water night and morning if you do soak them for this longer period.

> 50 g (2 oz) chickpeas, soaked for at least twelve
>   hours or overnight (or longer: see above)
> 1 garlic clove, crushed
> 30 ml (2 tbsp) lemon juice
> good pinch of salt
> black pepper
> 50 ml (2 fl oz) olive oil
> 100 ml (4 fl oz) water or orange juice
> 15 ml (1 tbsp) tahini

1. Transfer the soaked chickpeas and their liquid to a saucepan. Top up with fresh water, if necessary, to cover the chickpeas. Cover the pan and bring to the boil. Lower the heat and simmer for about two hours or until they are cooked, i.e. no longer hard. Drain.
2. Place the garlic, lemon juice, seasoning, oil and water in a blender. Liquidize, then gradually add the chickpeas, blending until smooth.
3. Add the tahini and liquidize again, adding a little extra liquid if the mixture is too dry.

Serves 2–4.

Main Meals

Caribbean Stew (**DF/GF**)
(from *The Neal's Yard Bakery Wholefood Cookbook* by Rachel Haigh

Quick and simple to make, this stew is given a truly Caribbean flavour by the creamed coconut and root ginger.

30 ml (2 tbsp) groundnut oil
1 large onion, finely chopped
1 red pepper, finely chopped
5 ml (1 tsp) grated root ginger
4 garlic cloves, crushed
1 small swede, cubed
1 small parsnip, cubed
1 large sweet potato, cubed
570 ml (1 pt) pineapple juice
30 ml (2 tbsp) tomato puree
60 ml (4 tbsp) creamed coconut
2.5–5 ml (½–1 tsp) chilli powder
salt and black pepper

1. Heat the oil in a medium-sized saucepan. Add the onion, red pepper, grated root ginger and crushed garlic. Sauté for five minutes, stirring occasionally, until the onion is soft.
2. Add the swede, parsnip and sweet potato to the saucepan and sauté for a further 3 minutes to seal in the flavours.
3. Add the pineapple juice, tomato puree, coconut, chilli powder and seasoning and simmer for 20 minutes or until the vegetables are cooked and tender.
4. Serve on a bed of brown rice.

Serves 6–8.

Aubergine Pie (*Melitzanpitta*) (**GF**)
(from *Greek Vegetarian Cookery* by Jack Santa Maria)

olive oil
1 onion, chopped
4 tomatoes, chopped
2–4 cloves garlic, finely chopped
1 tsp salt
½ tsp freshly ground black pepper
1 tsp basil
225 ml (8 fl oz) yoghurt

225 ml (8 fl oz) cottage or curd cheese
2 tsp sesame seeds
1 large aubergine
225 ml (8 fl oz) crumbled feta cheese
1 tbsp chopped parsley or coriander leaf

1. Preheat the oven to 350°F/180°C/Gas Mark 4.
2. Heat 2 tbsp of oil in a pan and fry the onion for 2 minutes. Add the tomatoes, garlic, salt, pepper and basil and cook together for 5 minutes.
3. Mix the yoghurt and cheese together with the sesame seeds.
4. Wash the aubergine and trim. Cut into thin slices. Heat half a cup of olive oil in a frying pan and fry the aubergine slices until golden. Remove and drain on absorbent paper.
5. Fill the bottom of a greased casserole or baking dish with some of the aubergine slices; cover with some of the tomato mixture and then with some of the yoghurt and cheese mixture. Put on another layer of aubergine, tomato and cheese as before. Cover with feta cheese. Bake in the oven until the top turns golden (30–40 minutes).
6. Serve garnished with the chopped herbs, with rice or baked potatoes and a green salad.

Serves 3.

Tofu Burgers (**DF/GF**)
(from *The Foodwatch Alternative Cookbook* by Honor J. Campbell

5 ml (1 tsp) olive oil
170 g (6 oz) leeks
110 g (4 oz) carrots
110 g (4 oz) mushrooms
1 tsp oregano
55g (2 oz) buckwheat or millet flakes
225 g (8 oz) tofu, thoroughly mashed
15 ml (2 tbsp) tahini
15 ml (2 tbsp) tamari

seasoning to taste
45 g (1½ oz) sesame seeds

1. Chop the leeks finely, coarsely grate the carrot and slice the mushrooms. Put the oil into a heavy based pan and heat. Add the prepared vegetables and sauté for about 8 minutes.
2. Remove from heat, add oregano, flakes, tofu, tahini, tamari and season with salt and pepper. Stir the mixture well and then leave to cool for a few minutes.
3. Divide the mixture into 8 portions and mould each one into a ball. Roll each ball in sesame seeds until well covered, and then flatten each ball into a burger shape with a potato masher or the palm of the hand. Grill or fry for about 5 minutes on each side.

Serves 4.

Swede and Orange Pie (DF/GF)
(from *The Neal's Yard Bakery Wholefood Cookbook* by Rachel Haigh)

Pureed swedes with a hint of orange and coconut make this an unusual dish.

30 ml (2 tbsp) soya oil
1 large onion, finely chopped
1 large red pepper, finely chopped
2 small turnips, finely chopped
1.5 tsp ground cinnamon
15 ml (1 tbsp) tomato puree
15 ml (1 tbsp) tamari
450 g (1 lb) courgettes, finely chopped
100 g (4 oz) mushrooms, finely chopped
salt and black pepper

For the topping:

1 kg (2 lb 3 oz) swedes, chopped
50 ml (2 fl oz) soya oil or 50 g (2 oz) butter

juice and grated rind of 1 orange
50 g (2 oz) desiccated coconut
salt and black pepper

1. Preheat the oven to 400°F/200°C/Gas Mark 6.
2. Boil the swedes for the topping for 10 minutes or steam them for 15 minutes, until tender.
3. Meanwhile, heat 30 ml (2 tbsp) oil in a medium-sized saucepan and add the onion, red pepper and turnips. Add the cinnamon, tomato puree and tamari and cook gently. Add the courgettes and mushrooms to the saucepan. Cook for a further 8–10 minutes or until the vegetables are tender. Season to taste.
4. By now the swedes should be ready. Drain well. Make the rest of the topping: add the oil, orange juice and rind and coconut to the swedes and blend to a smooth puree in a blender or with a potato masher. Season to taste.
5. Put the vegetables into an overproof dish and spread the swedes over the top. Bake for 20 minutes until cooked through. Serve immediately with a crisp green salad.

Serves 6.

Puddings, Cakes, Sweets and Biscuits

Strawberry Mousse (**DF/GF**)
(from *The Neal's Yard Bakery Wholefood Cookbook* by Rachel Haigh)

This mousse is made without eggs or dairy produce, but it wonderfully rich and creamy. You will need a blender.

570 ml (1 pt) unsweetened soya milk
15 ml (1 tbsp) agar-agar flakes
about 225 g (8 oz) strawberries, hulled
15 ml (1 tbsp) maple syrup

1. Pour the soya milk into a saucepan and add the agar-agar flakes. Bring to the boil and simmer for 5 minutes, stirring occasionally.

2. Pour the soya milk and agar-agar into a blender. Add the strawberries and the maple syrup and blend for 2–3 minutes until smooth.
3. Pour the mousse into a serving bowl or individual dishes and chill in the refrigerator for at least four hours.
4. Decorate with fresh strawberries before serving.

Serves 4.

Nerissa's chocolate (or carob) cake (DF/GF)

> 200 g (7 oz) rice flour
> gluten-free baking powder
> 30 ml (2 tbsp) cocoa or carob powder
> lashing of runny honey
> 125 ml (¼ pt) safflower oil
> 125 ml (¼ pt) soya milk
> 2 eggs

1. Preheat oven to 375°F/190°C/Gas Mark 5.
2. Put all ingredients in a mixer and blend well. The mixture will be runny.
3. Pour into two sandwich tins and bake for 35 minutes.
4. When cool, spread with Whole Earth Lime Spread (or whipped cream if dairy-free not desired).

Chocolate cake (DF/GF)
(from Berrydales newsletter, June 1994 – see 'Suppliers' under Useful Addresses in Appendix)

> 75 g (3 oz) dairy-free margarine
> 250 g (9 oz) dark muscovado sugar
> 60 ml (4 tbsp) gluten-free cocoa powder
> 3 eggs
> 100 g (4 oz) ground rice or rice flour
> 75 g (3 oz) ground almonds
> 1 tsp gluten-free baking powder

1. Preheat oven to 350°F/180°C/Gas Mark 4. Line a 20 cm (8 in) tin with greaseproof paper.

2. Beat together the fat and the sugar till light and fluffy.
3. Bring 100 ml (3 oz) water to the boil, pour on to the cocoa, mix well, then beat into the creamed mixture.
4. Beat in the eggs, adding a spoonful of rice flour with each.
5. Mix the baking powder into the remaining rice flour and ground almonds and fold into the mixture.
6. Spoon the mixture into the tin and bake in the oven for approximately 35 minutes or till the cake is firm to the touch. Cool on a wire rack before cutting.

Millet and Peanut Cookies (**DF/GF**)
(from *The Cranks Receipe Book* by David Canter, Kay Canter and Daphne Swann)

> 60 ml (4 tbsp) oil
> ¼ tsp salt
> 1 egg
> 75 g (3 oz) raw brown sugar
> 100 g (4 oz) ground peanuts
> 75 g (3 oz) raisins
> 100 g (4 oz) millet flakes

1. Preheat oven to 350°F/180°C/Gas Mark 4.
2. Lightly whisk together the oil, sugar, salt and eggs. Stir in the remaining ingredients until well blended. Roll the mixture into 10 balls. Place on a lightly greased baking sheet. Press each one down to flatten slightly.
3. Bake in the oven for about 15 minutes, until golden. Allow to cool on the baking sheet for a few minutes before transferring to a wire tray.

Brown Rice Digestive Biscuits (**DF/GF**)
(from *The Foodwatch Alternative Cookbook* by Honor J. Campbell)

> 110 g (4 oz) brown rice flour
> ¼ level tsp salt
> ½ level tsp gluten-free baking powder
> 45 g (1½ oz) dairy-free margarine

30 g (1 oz) sugar or 15 g (½ oz) fructose
45 ml (3 tbsp) goat's, sheep's or soya milk

1. Preheat oven to 375°F/190°C/Gas Mark 5.
2. Sieve together flour, salt and baking powder into a bowl. Rub in margarine and add sugar or fructose.
3. Mix to a stiff paste with milk. Turn on to a lightly floured surface and knead well. Roll out thinly.
4. Cut into rounds with 6 cm (2½ in) biscuit-cutter. Transfer on to a greased baking tray and prick well.
5. Bake for 12–15 minutes. Transfer to a wire rack to cool. Store in an airtight tin.

Potato Shortbread (DF/GF)
(from *The Foodwatch Alternative Cookbook* by Honor J. Campbell)

170 g (6 oz) potato flour
110 g (4 oz) dairy-free margarine
55 g (2 oz) sugar
85 g (3 oz) ground almonds or cashews

1. Preheat oven to 350°F/180°C/Gas Mark 4.
2. Beat margarine until soft and creamy. Add other ingredients and work until a ball of dough is formed. Put into a greased 18–20 cm (7–8 in) round sandwich tin and press down evenly. Prick all over and bake for 35–40 minutes or until lightly golden brown. Cut into 8 wedges.

Fruit and Nut Chews (DF/GF)

100 g (4 oz) raisins
100 g (4 oz) stoned dates
100 g (4 oz) walnuts
50 g (2 oz) dessicated coconut

1. Using a mincer fitted with a coarse blade, or a blender, mince or blend the raisins, dates and walnuts together.
2. Add the coconut and work the mixture with the fingertips until it binds.
3. Form into thin rolls and cut into bite-size pieces.

Carob 'Fudge' (GF)
(from *The Cranks Receipe Book* by David Canter, Kay Canter and
Daphne Swann)

> 50 g (2 oz) butter or margarine
> 25 g (1 oz) carob powder
> 50 g (2 oz) clear honey
> 25 g (1 oz) soya flour
> 75 g (3 oz) ground almonds
> 5 ml (1 tsp) vanilla essence
> 25 g (1 oz) almonds, ground or chopped finely

1. Cream the butter and carob powder until well mixed. Add the honey, soya flour, ground almonds and vanilla and mix thoroughly.
2. Sprinkle the ground almonds on a clean, dry working surface and shape the 'fudge' into a roll, coating it with the almonds.
3. Cut into a bite-sized pieces. Keep in the fridge until required.

Variation: for sesame 'fudge', replace 25 g (1 oz) ground almonds with 25 g toasted sesame seeds.

Useful Miscellaneous Recipes

Dairy-free Mayonnaise (DF/GF)
(from *The Neal's Yard Bakery Wholefood Cookbook* by Rachel
Haigh)

> 100 ml (4 fl oz) soya milk
> 60 ml (4 tbsp) lemon juice
> 10 ml (2 tsp) mustard powder
> 10 ml (2 tsp) finely chopped mixed herbs or
> 5 ml (1 tsp) dried herbs
> salt and black pepper
> 200–300 ml (7–11 fl oz) soya oil

1. Put the soya milk, lemon juice, mustard powder, herbs and seasoning in a blender. Liquidize until smooth.

2. Gradually add the oil, with the blender still running, until you have a thick consistency.

Makes about 425 ml (¾ pint). Keep in fridge.

Cornmeal Yorkshire Pudding (**DF/GF**)
(from *Good Food, Gluten Free* by Hilda Cherry Hills)

>112 ml (8 fl oz) cornmeal
>1 tsp salt
>½ tsp marjoram (optional)
>450 ml (¾ pint) milk or soya milk
>4 eggs, beaten
>1 tsp oil

1. Preheat oven to 350°F/180°C/Gas Mark 4.
2. Make paste from cornmeal, salt, marjoram and a quarter of the milk. Heat rest of milk in top of double boiler on direct heat. When it boils, add cornmeal paste. Stir until smooth. Place over hot water in double boiler. Cover. Cook gently until all liquid is absorbed. Remove.
3. When lukewarm, blend in eggs.
4. Oil large baking pan or individual ones, placed in preheated oven.
5. Pour in mixture to half full. Bake for 10 minutes.
6. Remove. Dot with remainder of oil. Return to oven and bake for another 15 minutes.

The following two sauces are made without flour of any kind.

Foam White Sauce (**DF/GF**)
(from *Good Food, Gluten Free* by Hilda Cherry Hills)

This sauce can be used for vegetables instead of standard white sauce.

>2 egg whites, beaten to a peak
>pinch of salt
>onion juice to taste

45 ml (3 tbsp) soya milk
chopped chives or parsley

1. Sprinkle salt into beaten egg white and mix in onion juice.
2. Gradually pour on the hot soya milk while beating well until it thickens.
3. Add chives or parsley.

Golden Cheese Sauce (**GF**)
(from *Good Food, Gluten Free* by Hilda Cherry Hills)

Serve this sauce with vegetables, fish, hot hard-boiled eggs etc.

2 egg yolks
60 ml (4 tbsp) finely grated cheese
salt to taste
30 ml (2 tbsp) butter

1. Beat the egg yolks with grated cheese and salt.
2. Melt the butter in top of double boiler or bowl over pan containing boiling water; add egg and cheese mixture and stir until it has thickened enough. Thin with a little milk if necessary.

Mock Cream (**DF/GF**)
(from *The Foodwatch Alternative Cookbook* by Honor J. Campbell)

1 level tbsp arrowroot flour
75 ml (5 tbsp) cold water
45 g (1½ oz) dairy-free margarine
sweetener to taste

1. Place arrowroot in a saucepan and add water, stirring all the time.
2. Heat and stir until the mixture thickens. Beat until smooth, then put in a basin and leave until completely cold.
3. Add margarine and beat well.

4. Sweeten to taste and continue to beat until fluffy. Use within 2 days.

Nut Cream (**DF/GF**)

> 110 g (4 oz) cashews or blanched almonds
> honey or maple syrup to taste
> 90 ml (6 tbsp) water

Blend or grind nuts to fine powder. Add rest of ingredients and blend until smooth and creamy. Chill in fridge.

Psychological Treatments of IBS

Brenda Toner and Claire Rutter

Most people, if asked what they thought psychotherapeutic techniques involved, and how helpful they were, would probably answer that they are wholly focused on events which happened in childhood, and of use only in dealing with mental disorders. In fact, psychotherapy involves helping people with all sorts of problems, by 'talking treatments'. There are various different techniques, but they share the basic method of the therapist and the patient talking about events, thoughts and feelings that matter to that individual, for example their problems, their everyday lives, their worries and fears. The therapist then pursues these discussions with the individual to gain a greater understanding of their problems and how they could be alleviated.

How Can Psychotherapy Help People with Physical Symptoms, such as those in IBS?

Whatever your view is of why you have IBS, psychotherapy may be able to help you come to terms with your problem, and in some cases may even help to reduce your symptoms, or provide you with some coping strategies to deal with them.

Researchers have found that what distinguishes IBS patients from people without IBS is the reactivity of the colon to environmental events. The changes in bowel activity associated with the disorder have been shown to be associated with heightened arousal of emotions such as anxiety and anger. Since it seems that there is a link between IBS and stress, and since it is virtually impossible to avoid stressful situations, it makes sense to consider ways in which you might improve the way you cope with stress: this is where a psychotherapist can help.

Also, if your symptoms *are* associated with psychological factors, then a therapist will also be able to construct a programme of treatment that could help. Some of these factors are discussed later in this chapter.

How Successful is Psychotherapy in Treating IBS?

Assessing trials of psychotherapy for IBS patients is not straightforward, given the varied nature of people's symptoms, and the lack of carefully controlled studies in this area. However, some research results do suggest that psychotherapeutic treatment may be beneficial.

In one experiment conducted in 1985, thirty-three IBS patients were given either medical or psychological treatments, after having six weeks with no treatment. It was found that the psychological treatments helped lower distress by reducing both anxiety and IBS symptoms. Another team of researchers gave fifty-one IBS patients medical care and fifty others short-term psychotherapy plus medical care: after treatment, those who had had psychotherapy had improved, feeling less pain and less physical symptoms. This improvement was still evident one year after treatment. In another trial, patients were given either medical treatment alone or medical treatment plus psychotherapy. Three months after treatment, the researchers found a significant improvement in the psychotherapy group on self-ratings of diarrhoea and pain, compared to their original condition, although no improvement in constipation. They stated that psychological treatment is feasible and effective in two-thirds of patients who do not respond to standard medical treatment.

While these studies are promising in that they show that psychological interventions might be useful for people with IBS, much of the research in this area suffers from problems which limit interpretation of the findings: for example, in some studies the therapeutic techniques were not adequately described or monitored; and many people refused to take part in the experiments, which limits the generalizability of the results. However, the fact that the majority of studies were not carefully controlled and monitored does not make them worthless. Many people believe they have been helped by psychotherapy; and it has been claimed that psycho-therapy can lead to a significant improvement, both in symptoms and in accompanying mood states, and that these improvements can be maintained for several months at least.

What to Expect from Psychotherapy

Therapists use different methods in their attempts to help you overcome your symptoms. There are various basic types of approach, and each therapist will also have his or her preferred techniques and style. In the rest of this chapter, we will describe the different techniques you may encounter if you try psychotherapy, focusing in particular on the two main types of psychotherapy used in treating IBS: cognitive-behavioral therapy and exploratory psychotherapy. Whatever the particular aproach used, most therapists will offer an initial assessment, at which you will be asked about your symptoms, relationships, family history, employment and so on. At this stage, you and the therapist can negotiate what treatment entails and what you hope to achieve – the 'treatment goals'. Also, you can discuss how long you are likely to be in therapy, and, if the treatment is private, the actual cost. At all times therapists should ensure confiden-tiality. If you are having therapy under the NHS, you may be asked for details of your GP, and your therapist will usually notify him or her should you engage in treatment. If you are paying for private treatment this may not happen; you should ask your therapist his or her policy on this point.

Group Psychotherapy or Individual Psychotherapy?

Most of the techniques mentioned in this chapter can be conducted either in groups or individually. Which is chosen depends on the patient's preference, or sometimes on which is available in the patient's locality.

Group psychotherapy is typically conducted with a small number of individuals, usually between about six and twelve, who all have the same problem(s). The advantage of the group approach is that the individual can derive comfort and support from observing that others have similar experiences. Also, in the case of IBS sufferers for whom the condition is a major hindrance to social life, it may provide the opportunity to make friends with people in a similar situation, without the embarrassment of either hiding or explaining the problem. The advantage of individual therapy on the other hand, is that the specific techniques are tailored more specifically to the individual's individual needs and goals.

Psychodrama

The earliest use of the group process in psychotherapy can be credited to the Austrian Jacob Moreno (1910), who combined dramatic and therapeutic techniques to create what he called 'psychodrama'. He conducted his therapy on stage, with people in the group playing key figures in the patient's life. He would also instruct patients to reverse roles to gain a greater awareness of how other people saw them. This may seem a strange method, but many have claimed that role-playing techniques offer patients valuable insights and feedback that help them to achieve a better understanding of themselves.

A Swedish study looked at the effectiveness of psychodrama and relaxation training in the treatment of IBS. Patients were invited to have conversations with their own stomach or gut, played by another group member. The aim here was to make the participants aware of the interplay between emotions and bodily symptoms. After the initial treatment, both symptom levels and anxiety levels dropped; however, symptom levels tended to rise again after three years.

Cognitive-Behavioral Group Therapy

Cognitive behaviour therapists believe that what you think about the things that you do, and the reasons behind your actions, are as important as your behaviour. The aim of this particular therapy is to modify unhelpful or damaging beliefs as a means of overcoming problem behaviour. A team of researchers led by Brenda Toner in Toronto has recently completed a study investigating the use of cognitive-behavioral group therapy in treating IBS: this study will be used here as an illustration of the cognitive-behavioral method in practice.

The group consisted of six IBS sufferers, who all started and finished treatment at the same time, and one therapist. Group sessions took place weekly for twelve weeks, each session lasting ninety minutes. One treatment session took place before the beginning of the first group session, in order to begin teaching people about cognitive-behavioral therapy, to establish initial rapport with each IBS sufferer and to identify treatment goals.

At each group session, there was a predetermined agenda set by the therapist as well as individual agenda items chosen by each group member for that session, for example dealing with a stressful situation at work. The following items were always included in the group agenda:

- a progressive relaxation exercise to begin the session (this involves tightening and relaxing each muscle group);
- indivudal members' agenda items (e.g. each member may report on something they want the group's help with);
- individual members' reactions to the previous session;
- members' own reports of their mental and physical state and any other significant events during the week;
- therapist's review of previous session's self-help assignments (e.g. the outcome of homework tasks);
- introduction of any new cognitive theory or technique for that session;
- discussion of selected individual agenda items (e.g. individuals may agree to try out a new way of thinking about a problem or to carry out a particular task);
- new self-help assignments;
- summary of session;
- individuals' reactions to the current session.

The Roles of Therapist and Patient

It is not surprising that people with IBS, who are suffering physical symptoms and pain, may interpret referrals to psychologists or psychiatrists as insulting and personally diminishing. The critical challenge to the therapist is to counter the implication that IBS symptoms are imaginary or caused by underlying mental problems. Only when this task is successfully addressed is a therapeutic alliance possible.

The therapist giving treatment does not consider him or herself an expert on your situation; on the contrary, they see you as the best person to evaluate your own experience and want to enable you to be a 'personal scientist'. Some IBS sufferers see themselves as victims of their disease or as devoid of control over their bodily reactions; and they may see that stress as something which happens to them from the outside, over which they have little control. These beliefs need to be evaluated in the open.

An attempt to encourage you to be a personal scientist involves three steps. The first step is to encourage you to gather information about your thoughts and emotions in stressful situations. The second step involves asking you to examine whether there is any relationship between these pieces of information (therapists can be particularly helpful in this phase by pointing out possible connections between thoughts and feelings, e.g. the thought may be 'I am upset' and the feeling may be 'sad' or 'tearful'). Step three involves helping you to become aware of the beliefs which you have and to examine the extent to which the data you collect (your beliefs) are supported or not supported.

An example might be someone who believes that showing a need for emotional contact with others or giving overt displays of affection are signs of weakness. Gathering information may involve asking other people how they feel about the expression of emotion, examining the patterns of emotional expression in the family or recalling instances when you felt good about other people expressing emotion to you. In this way, feedback from others is used to challenge some of the beliefs you might have about expressing emotion as signs of weakness.

The value of the therapist taking this stance is that he or she avoids being in a position of telling you that he or she knows what is best for you. This may appear difficult at first: you may want the therapist to find the solution for you. At the same time, however, the therapist can reassure you that this process has been found to be helpful in the past, and that there is good reason to believe that it will continue to be helpful in your case. The questions asked by the therapist are phrased in a manner requiring judgement on the part of the IBS sufferer and evincing respect for his or her beliefs. The therapist does not generally assume the role of expert, but rather assumes that of facilitator.

This approach establishes the collaborative relationship that is central to cognitive-behavioral intervention. Goals (what you want to achieve) are mutually agreed upon and are developed in consideration of the individual's current status, his or her particular strengths, limitations or disabilities, and the more general goals for treatment. The result of this negotiation process must be the establishment of goals that the individual feels are obtainable as well as personally relevant to his or her particular needs.

Examples of Common Themes in Cognitive-Behavioral Sessions

On the basis of previous research, we feel that there are several themes common to many individuals who come to us with IBS.

Thoughts, feelings and gastrointestinal symptoms

In this type of therapy interactions between thoughts (cognitions), emotions and gastrointestinal symptoms are explored. In particular, the cognitive-behavioral model is used to highlight how certain thoughts and underlying beliefs may lead to increased attention to bodily sensations and increased arousal and heightened sensitivity to pain and other gastrointestinal symptoms. The daily record of dysfunctional thoughts (i.e. thoughts which do not serve a useful purpose) is introduced and used during sessions to identify and alter dysfunctional thoughts.

Coping with stress and anxiety

Stressful situations are identified and coping strategies dicussed; anxiety hierarchies are introduced. To construct an anxiety hierarchy, you are asked to identify situations that you find most stressful and then to rank according to the degree of anxiety they produce on a scale of 1–100 points. When the ranking process is complete, specific anxiety-reducing methods of treatment are given. In addition, thoughts relating to these situations are identified, challenged and modified throughout the course of treatment.

Assertiveness

Assertiveness is defined as the direct, honest and appropriate expression of opinions, beliefs, needs and feelings. Previous research and clinical experience have suggested that people with gastrointestinal disorders have particular difficulty in being assertive. Training and homework assignments are especially directed at challenging the underlying thoughts and beliefs that inhibit expressions of your opinions, needs and feelings.

Anger

Techniques are introduced which help you to identify how reactive or easily irritated you are in various situations. The interplay among thoughts, anger, physiological arousal, non-assertive behaviour and symptoms is highlighted.

Social approval

In cognitive-behavioral group work with IBS sufferers, assumptions frequently centre on three major issues: heightened need for social approval (wanting others to like you); perfectionism (the need for things to be perfect or 'right'); and the need for control (or certainty). Thoughts and underlying beliefs concerning a heightened need for approval from others are examined in the light of gastrointestinal symptoms. The relationships between the need to please others, difficulties with and fears of doing something publicly unacceptable are identified and challenged.

Perfectionism

Thoughts about appearing less than perfect are identified and challenged. Cognitive and behaviour techniques are directed at working with group members to change extreme, all-or-nothing attitudes about being perfect.

Control

Techniques and assignments are used to demonstrate the limitations of the control ideal. Some people with gastrointestinal disorders respond to their symptoms by trying to control aspects of their environment that may be associated with symptoms: this then paradoxically limits their freedom, that is, has the opposite effect to that they intended. By trying to exercise control and achieve certainty in all situations, people lose opportunities to collect evidence that they can handle situations.

The Final Session
This session is spent primarily discussing progress to date towards treatment goals. Cognitive and behavioral strategies are reviewed in light of how you have been able to use them in daily living. Particular emphasis is placed on their continued use once treatment has ended.

How Successful is this Approach?
The results given here are only preliminary, as we have not yet obtained follow-up data, but nevertheless look promising. We found that IBS sufferers who had cognitive-behavioral group treatment experienced a lessening of depression, while sufferers who had conventional medical treatment actually had more depressive symptoms.

We asked IBS sufferers to fill out a daily diary on their IBS symptoms for two weeks before therapy, two weeks following therapy and again for two weeks six months after the therapy had ended. We found that IBS sufferers in the cognitive-behavioral group had less bloating following therapy compared to a group which only received information on IBS, e.g. the causes, symptoms and possible treatments (This latter group was called the 'psychoeducational' group.) There was also a group who had medical treatment only. On a combined measure of diarrhoea and/or constipation symptoms, there was improvement in both the cognitive-behavioral and the psychoeducational groups compared with the group given only conventional medical therapy.

IBS sufferers in the cognitive-behavioral group found therapy to be more effective for them than sufferers in the other two groups (psychoeducational and medical). Specifically, members in the cognitive-behavioral group reported significantly stronger identification with the following statements:

- 'I am better able to cope with my symptoms as a result of participating in the group;'
- 'Participation in the group has helped me to cope better in other areas of my life that have turned out to be in crisis;'
- 'My IBS symptoms have improved as a result of participating in the group;'
- 'I look more on the positive side of things as a result of participating in the group;'
- 'My level of confidence has increased as a result of participating in the group;'
- 'I found the group to be more helpful than I had expected.'

Exploratory Psychotherapy

The principle underlying this method is that your physical and psychological problems arise from disturbances in significant personal relationships. Improvement in your interpersonal relationships should therefore result in a reduction of your symptoms. The creation of an interpersonal relationship with the therapist, who adopts a warm, friendly manner and expresses sympathy and understanding, allows your problems to be revealed, explored and understood.

The following outline of the different types of sessions used is based on the practice of a group in Manchester led by Drs Guthrie and Creed.

The Initial Session

The first session is quite long, lasting approximately three hours. The goals of this first session include establishing a firm working relationship between you and the therapist, and helping you to make a link between physical symptoms and psychological processes. The strategies used include: exploring irrational fears you may have about therapy; taking a detailed history of your symptoms; exploring in depth the personal meaning of your symptoms and their effect on you; assessing your early life experiences and contact with sickness. Specific techniques used include the use of statements rather than questions, and specific use by the therapist of bowel-related metaphors (e.g. 'full of shit', 'bunged up').

The Intermediate Sessions

The main goal of the intermediate sessions is to work on the problem areas identified in the initial session. Strategies include exploring further the development of symptoms; identifying reasons for the continuance of symptoms; and linking interpersonal difficulties outside therapy to interpersonal processes in the session. In addition to the techniques used in the opening session, the therapist will introduce the use of bowel charts to link bowel disturbance to interpersonal conflict.

The Final Session

The goals of the final session include the identification of positive changes that have occurred during therapy, and consideration of how these can be maintained after therapy has finished, and the exploration of any negative changes or feelings.

Using this model of exploratory psychotherapy, Drs Guthrie and Creed found that, compared to a control group, sufferers showed significant improvements on ratings of diarrhoea and abdominal pain, and this led to reduced health care utilization for one year following therapy.

Stress Management Techniques

This section focuses on some specific techniques that psychotherapists may use in approaching the problems of IBS sufferers. Since more than half of patients with IBS report that their symptoms are made worse by stress, and more than half report an acute episode of stress preceding the first onset of symptoms, it is not surprising that psychotherapists have focused in particular on developing techniques for managing stress.

Arousal Reduction Training/Relaxation Training

The aim of this technique is to reduce and control emotional arousal and anxiety, using progressive muscle relaxation training, non-specific biofeedback training (discussed below), autogenic training or meditation. It is important to realize that all mental health professionals (psychologists, psychiatrists, nurses and social workers as well as therapists) may use these techniques.

Progressive muscle relaxation training is the most commonly used arousal reduction technique. The aim is to tense and then relax each major group of muscles in turn, while concentrating on the sensation within. This is an easy exercise that you can practise at home; cassette tapes with specific exercises recorded on them are available.

Some investigators have reported good results in IBS patients with these exercises alone. One psychologist used relaxation training together with brief psychotherapy in twenty IBS patients and reported significant reductions in psychiatric symptoms (depression and anxiety) as well as modest reductions in bowel symptoms.

Self-Control

This technique works by the therapist getting the patient to recognize the onset of tension and then using arousal reduction techniques to guard off undue stress.

Biofeedback

This is a more technological method of stress management, and requires patients to be given information about their bodies which is not normally available to them. With the aid of electronic instruments they can either see or hear what is going on in their bodies; by observing how physical reactions are triggered, it is hoped that they can learn to control their bodies even when the amplifying instrument is removed.

Two types of biofeedback have been used in treating IBS patients, specific and non-specific. Non-specific biofeedback involves the use of the technique to teach relaxation, whereas specific biofeedback involves feedback on bowel motility itself to teach the patient to inhibit the response.

One psychologist applied biofeedback successfully on IBS patients: he used an electronic stethoscope to amplify bowel sounds and trained his patients alternately to increase and decrease the volume of sound. He reported that all five patients were able to learn this response, and that all five experienced symptomatic improvement.

Self-Regulation

This is a method of self-control developed by Japanese researchers. The patient is instructed to get into a state of relaxed alertness, achieved by focusing attention on their breathing and body warmth (active thinking is discouraged). The patient sits upright, with a straight spine, palms placed flat on the thighs, legs comfortably apart with the feet touching the floor (ideally the patient should be barefoot). The patient is told to breathe gently, inhaling through the nose, and exhaling through the mouth. The patient is then instructed to say to him/herself 'I am feeling relaxed.' Then the treatment begins. Each stage must be mastered before the next stage begins.

In stage 1, the therapist draws the patient's attention to the warmth of the palms on the thighs. This stage usually takes around five minutes to complete, but obviously it varies with individual experience. In stage 2, the warmth of the hands is suggested to spread to the forearms. In stage 3, the patient becomes aware of how their feet are touching the floor, and then focuses on the warmth in their feet. In stage 4, the warmth of the feet is suggested to spread to the legs. In stage 5, the patient focuses on the coolness of the forehead region (sometimes this is achieved by patients suggesting to themselves that the forehead region feels refreshed). In stage 6, the control of the internal organs is practised. This is usually achieved by moving one hand (either one) from the thighs to the abdomen, and then suggesting to oneself: 'My abdomen is warm.' In practised patients, stages 3–6 will take around five to ten minutes.

This particular technique was used to treat a teenager with IBS, and it was claimed that it improved his diarrhoea.

One research team evaluated this treatment and concluded that those IBS patients who were less anxious at the beginning of the treatment were more likely to show a significant clinical improvement. However, it was predicted that the more anxious patient simply needs longer, more intensive treatment.

Systematic Desensitization

If you have symptoms of IBS that always seem to flare up in certain non-stressful situations, some psychologists would say that you have become 'conditioned' to respond thus. This means that you have learned to pair a certain situation (or behaviour) with the worsening of your symptoms. This would happen, for example, if your symptoms were bad during a particular non-stressful situation in the past, and you have tended to worry that they will worsen again if the situation is repeated: so, whenever you do encounter a similar situation (e.g. a car journey), you automatically feel worse. Once this connection is established such sufferers tend to avoid these seemingly non-stressful situations, and so the connection becomes stronger.

In the treatment of this particular problem therapists use a technique called systematic desensitization, which is designed to produce a decrease in anxiety associated with a feared situation (or object, or behaviour). This is achieved by using a gradual approach consisting of four basic steps. First, the patient learns to think of anxiety in terms of subjective units along a 100-point scale, where 100 is the situation that would create the most anxiety imaginable, and 0 is the calmest. For example, 100 might be being stuck in a traffic jam on a motorway with no services, and 0 would be thinking about going on a very short car journey with toilets at either end. Secondly, the patient would be given relaxation training (the exact technique used will vary between therapists). Thirdly, the patient and the therapist work together to produce an anxiety hierarchy, ranking situations according to their anxiety-involving properties for that individual. Fourthly, the patient progressively imagines being in each of the scenes of the hierarchy, starting from 0, while trying to remain relaxed. The patient will not move on to the next scene/situation until they are able to visualize the previous one without feeling any anxiety. This stage will vary in duration for different individuals, and will progress until the patient reaches the top of their own unique hierarchy. It is hoped that a previously feared situation will then be paired with an automatic relaxation response.

Combining Medical and Psychotherapeutic Treatments

For a long time IBS treatment was primarily medical, based on drugs and diet therapy, both of which provide only minimal relief from symptoms. More recently, published research has included multicomponent treatment packages or combined techniques, including various combinations of cognitive-behavioural, relaxation, psychodynamic and biofeedback approaches. For example, one team of researchers devised a combined treatment programme for IBS patients which included: education about normal bowel functioning; progressive relaxation; thermal biofeedback; and cognitive techniques for coping with stress. Those patients taking drugs for their condition, and following special diets, continued to do so. The subjects found significant reductions in abdominal pain and diarrhoea. It was reported that similar results were achieved when this combined technique was conducted in one-to-one therapy, but that some patients expressed particular satisfaction with the group format, through finding that they are not alone with IBS. (However, the cognitive treatment was found to be more successful in individual therapy, where each patient's needs and problems could be addressed in more depth.) Moreover, 57 per cent of the patients treated in this way were still experiencing clinical improvement in their condition two years later.

It is best to look upon psychotherapy as an addition to, or integrated with, medical treatment, not as an alternative to it. If you believe that you might benefit from psychotherapy, go ahead and give it a try. And remember, any treatment will be more effective if you believe in it, and are motivated to stick with it. The expectation that one will get better, the development of a trusting relationship with a therapist, and a strong desire that it will happen are essential ingredients of hope, and hope can have a powerful impact on our emotions and bodily responses.

Further Aspects of Psychological Interventions

One important area that needs to be developed and incorporated into work with IBS is an appreciation of the distress that is caused by living with a debilitating chronic illness which arouses little understanding or empathy, and with which considerable stigma is associated, with trivialization of the condition widespread on the part of both society in general and the medical system in particular. Another area that needs to be considered is the influence of gender on IBS. Despite the repeated documentation of a significant gender imbalance in sufferers from the condition, with three women to every man, little attention has been devoted to gender issues in either the conceptualization or the clinical management of IBS.

The Stigma Associated with Functional Somatic Syndromes

Nearly every medical specialty has identified a functional somatic syndrome (FSS). These syndromes are usually defined by physical symptoms unexplained by organic disease. The term 'functional' implies a disturbance of physiological function rather than anatomical structure; because of the stigma associated with the term, various alternative labels have been used to describe FSS, including 'somatic disorders', 'health anxiety', 'physical symptoms unexplained by organic disease', 'unexplained medical symptoms' and 'psychophysiological disorders'. Three of the most common functional somatic syndromes on which increased research and clinical attention has been targeted during the last decade are Irritable Bowel Syndrome (IBS), Chronic Fatigue Syndrome (CFS) and Fibromyalgia Syndrome (FS).

In western societies in general, and in medicine in particular, illness is either attributed to impersonal causes and viewed as an accident that befalls the patient as a victim, or is viewed as psychologically caused, and potentially under the person's voluntary control. Pejorative moral connotations therefore become attached to a functional somatic disorder, often leaving patients believing that their problems are due to a psychological or moral defect or weakness in themselves, and are being treated as 'not real'. Women are especially alive to the possibility that their symptoms are not taken seriously, because research has found that disorders disproportionately prevalent in women are often trivialized or described as psychological in origin. Unfortunately, 'trivial' and 'psychological' are often equated, and therefore sufferers may not want to discuss psychological factors in their illness since to do so seems to provide further evidence that health professionals are not taking their symptoms seriously. When individuals with FSS are referred to a mental health professional, they may come into the consultation with the belief that the therapist does not think their symptoms are 'real' or serious, but 'all in their head'. The therapeutic alliance cannot be established unless the reality of the symptoms is validated. Our group finds that a psychoeducational session focusing on the interplay among psychological, social and biological factors in illness is helpful early on in the treatment of FSS.

In the persistent search for organic causes, both patient and doctor become frustrated and the doctor–patient relationship is compromised. This can lead to various outcomes that serve further to heighten the sufferer's distress and fuel the vicious circle of perpetuating factors. Because you are understandably hypervigilant to any hint that medical specialists, friends, family, employer or society are not taking your symptoms seriously, you may become even more determined to find the medical cause to your very real pain and physical suffering. You may also experience added worry and self-doubt arising from the ambiguity of your illness. This lack of clarity in your experience may in turn heighten certain forms of behaviour, such as the rejection of any psychological influence in an effort to obtain medical and social validation for your suffering.

The Gender Issue in Therapy

It is important to consider issues of gender in therapy because research suggests that gender plays a role in influencing individuals' reactions to various situations, as well as how they perceive themselves and are perceived by others.

Several writers have suggested that in certain fundamental ways women experience a different social reality from that experienced by men. Accordingly, certain areas require added focus in therapy because of their relevance to women's social context. We have identified several salient areas in the lives of women who have received a diagnosis of IBS. These fall under two general themes: (1) history of sexual and physical abuse; and (2) areas that have been influenced by gender role socialization, including physical functioning and relationship issues concerning nurturance, assertion and pleasing others.

Physical and sexual abuse

One research team found that a history of sexual and physical abuse is a frequent, often undetected experience in women seen in gastroenterology clinics and is particularly common in patients with functional gastrointestinal disorders. Specifically, 44 per cent of a consecutive sample of 206 women seen in a referral-based gastroenterology practice had experienced sexual and/or physical abuse. Almost one-third of the abused patients had never discussed their experiences with anyone and only 17 per cent had informed their doctors. The same study also found that women with functional gastrointestinal disorders were significantly more likely than those with organic diseases to report forced intercourse, frequent physical abuse, incest, chronic or recurrent abdominal pain and more experience of surgery. Abused women were more likely than non-abused women to report pelvic pain, multiple somatic symptoms, more surgery and greater resort to health care. The frequency of abuse found in this study is similar to that reported in studies of women who suffer from chronic pelvic pain, but who are not found to have anything gynaecologically wrong with them upon laparoscopy. Other researchers also found that approximately three-quarters of female IBS patients had sexual disorders which may be related in part to findings of sexual abuse.

Hypervigilance and IBS

Researchers have identified common thoughts concerning body functioning in women clients. These frequently involve concerns over losing control, doing something socially unacceptable, appearing less than perfect, having something physically wrong with one's body and not being able to control bodily functions through thoughts or behaviour. A common phenomenon is a hypervigilance or hyperawareness of any notable body sensation, with corresponding hyperconcern over the potential meaning of that sensation. Men as well as women may be subject to developing these thoughts and attitudes; however, girls undergo a socialization process that is more likely to emphasize appearance, self-control and restraint in physical activity. For example, in regard to gastrointestinal functions, while belching and passing gas are not usually socially desirable in public for either sex, girls and women are socialized into believing that these bodily functions are especially not 'ladylike' (e.g. 'belching and farting' contests are less frequent among female than among male adolescents). Moreover, bowel function is considered a taboo subject in 'polite' conversation, and talking about associated symptoms is viewed as lacking in good taste, embarrassing and even shameful, especially for women.

Monitoring exacerbates symptoms

Many IBS patients report that their fear of experiencing bowel symptoms in public places often exacerbates the symptoms themselves, resulting in further avoidance of public situations. Such avoidance can lead to personal and social isolation, another factor in the stress and depressed mood experienced by clients with a diagnosis of IBS. The following example of a 37-year-old office worker highlights the anxiety associated with bowel functioning:

'Whenever I went to the office dinners, I lived in fear for weeks thinking of all the excuses that I could make for not attending. For two days before, I would try to eat as little as possible with the hope that my bowels would not act up. I always arrived early at the restaurant to scout out the toilets so I could try to choose a seat as close as possible to the washroom so that I could sneak away as unobtrusively as possible should I need to use the washroom. During the meal I picked at the food but felt too anxious to eat anything. I was starving, but it was better than all the tumult that I could experience in my bowels when I ate in this situation. Every time my stomach rumbled I felt like crawling under the table.'

Most individuals with IBS are sensitive to any changes in their gastrointestinal system. Individuals who have experienced embarrassment because of IBS in social situations enter such situations highly attuned to any signs that might signal pain or dysfunction of the gut. Once any such change is noted, the focus on this is amplified and the individual begins to worry and become stressed.

The following is a useful behavioral intervention to give clients a greater sense of power over their symptoms. Clients are instructed to monitor their symptoms every two or three minutes when they are experiencing them, rating them on a severity scale of one to ten. On another occasion when they are experiencing symptoms, they are instructed to try to focus on something that is not connected with their pain (looking out of the window, for example). After this, in the debriefing session, it is useful to ask how their symptoms were affected by the two different focus strategies.

Nurturance

Clients with unexplained medical symptoms (including IBS) are often quite surprised to realize how poorly they nurture themselves. It has been suggested that these patients often go out of their way to help others, but do not take time to nurture themselves. Women with IBS often express pride in their ability to give practical and emotional support to their partners and children at home and to their colleagues at work. Neglecting herself can often mean that a woman in this situation is not attuned to her own psychological and emotional needs; however, a woman with severe IBS symptoms is forced by her gastrointestinal problems to be aware of her physical difficulties. Consequently, she is hindered in being aware of the connection between her own self-neglect, the resulting stress and its impact on her symptoms.

It can be seen that part of this cycle of denying one's need for self-nurturance and internalizing the belief that women gain pleasure from nurturing others is that a woman under stress may attempt to alleviate her stress by being even more nurturing of others. For women with IBS, this can be a potentially unhealthy coping strategy because these women often report that the more nurturing they are of others, the more nurturance is expected of them. This further self-neglect may result in greater personal stress as well as increased severity in associated bowel symptoms.

Non-assertion and need for approval

Gender role socialization has encouraged girls and women to be non-assertive, putting others' needs before their own, not expressing anger and being attuned to other people's feelings. One consequence of this is that women have problems with anger and assertion more often than men. Common underlying beliefs that have been identified in women clients are central themes with women diagnosed with IBS. These include 'I don't have a right to push my opinion on others,' 'It's better to please others and selfish to please myself,' 'Others always come first,' and 'It's not ladylike to raise your voice or show anger.'

When individuals feel powerless or their needs are not being met, angry feelings will be evoked. In the absence of 'permission' to express these needs directly, women are likely to be more critical and self-blaming. Moreover, when women do behave in an assertive manner, it is often perceived by others as aggressive or inappropriate, again on the basis of gender role expectations. The relationships between the need to please others, the expression of anger, assertion difficulties and self-esteem need to be explored.

These empirical findings and clinical observations have implications for both the assessment and treatment of individuals with IBS. Health-care providers and researchers alike need to become more aware of factors such as the stigmatization, trivialization and shame that have been associated with IBS and the influence of gender role socialization, and to integrate this awareness into therapies.

We need to challenge society's negative view of bowel functioning. This is likely to be quite a struggle, since the stigma associated with 'the bowels' is very strong in our society; but it is worth 'coming out of the closet' for, until this happens, many people with IBS will continue to suffer a debilitating and often misunderstood illness in silence.

5

The Treatment of IBS
by Hypnotherapy

*Elizabeth E. Taylor**

We have all heard of hypnosis – but how many of us have any accurate idea of its use? Old films and even modern cartoons leave us with images of swinging watches and domineering voices commanding the subject to 'Look into my eyes' and 'Go to sleep ... sleep ... sleep ...' Equally worrying are the misconceptions created by the stage hypnotist who seems to be able, by the mere click of his fingers, to 'compel' his volunteers to caress a mop head, believing it to be a loved one's hair, or to cluck like a chicken or bark like a dog – all in the name of entertainment! These delusions give hypnosis a bad name. The stage hypnotist cleverly selects either exhibitionist or obedient 'volunteers' who enjoy playing the fool in public. The theatrical atmosphere and audience expectations do the rest. Further misconceptions arise from expressions such as 'putting someone under' and 'getting stuck in hypnosis', which encourage fears that the hypnotist will dominate the subject's mind.

All these notions are naturally off-putting, but none actually has anything to do with medical hypnosis, which for IBS sufferers is merely a tool to enable you to overcome the distressing symptoms that make your life a misery.

This chapter reviews information and research on the

---

* The author would like to thank her patients for allowing details of their cases to be published.

treatment of IBS with hypnotherapy. It will discuss both physical and emotional considerations and will outline the different approaches available to suit different individuals. A detailed account of what to expect in both 'gut-directed' and analytical hypnotherapy will be given. Case reports are included, with the permission of the patients concerned, to provide examples: the individuals' names have been altered to protect their identity. Suggested mechanisms by which hypnotherapy may benefit IBS sufferers are outlined, together with details of the availability and cost of this kind of treatment.

What is Hypnosis?

Hypnosis can be described as an altered state of conscious awareness. It is a natural state or relaxation, similar to daydreaming or the condition of complete absorption in an activity, such as reading, watching television, etc. You are aware and can hear people talking to you, but you remain entirely absorbed in what you are doing. In hypnosis the imagination rather than the intellect is active. There is no loss of control: you and the therapist form a team, and if you are unwilling to cooperate it is impossible for the therapist to effect a change. In the clinical setting, the hypnotherapist is unable to make you do or say anything you do not want to do or say. Nearly everyone can enter the hypnotic state. The depth of relaxation is irrelevant to a successful outcome, and it is usually the intelligent individual with a high motivation for change who achieves the best results.

What to Expect

During an initial consultation, you and your therapist will get to know one another; hypnosis is explained, and any worries you may have about treatment will be discussed. At the second visit hypnosis is induced. This involves listening to suggestions of deep relaxation – contrary to widespread belief, it does not involve unconsciousness and has nothing to do with sleep; you will be aware of what is said. Nevertheless you will allow yourself to enter an altered state of consciousness which is usually described as a very pleasant relaxing sensation. The induction of hypnosis itself can be very beneficial and, when combined with further suggestions specific to you, can be used to eliminate or alleviate many common problems. Hypnotherapy is not a miracle cure; rather it is a state of awareness that can be used for self-help. A strong commitment on the part of both you and your therapist is essential for a successful outcome.

Some people worry about remaining in hypnosis indefinitely, that is, about getting 'stuck' in the hypnotic state. This is in fact impossible: as with sleep or daydreaming, people emerge naturally from hypnosis, particularly if there is a need to do so.

Can Hypnosis Help People with IBS?

This question was addressed by Dr Peter Whorwell, a consultant physician in Manchester, who with his colleagues carried out a controlled trial on hypnotherapy and IBS in 1984. He selected thirty patients with severe symptoms of IBS who had failed to respond to other forms of treatment. These patients were randomly divided into two groups. One group received individual half-hour sessions of hypnosis over a three-month period; the second group acted as a 'control'. This second group was given the same amount of time and attention as the hypnosis group, but without the hypnosis sessions. Patients discussed thir symptoms and described any stressful incidents in their lives which they thought may have contributed to their bowel problem. They were also given a 'placebo', i.e. tablets which they believed would help their condition but in fact contained no medication (sugar pills). The idea behind this was to control for the 'placebo effect'. Very often, if a person expects a treatment to work it does: the effect of the mind on the body is quite remarkable. If the hypnosis group improved beyond the level attributable to the placebo effect, this would constitute good evidence that the hypnotherapy itself was causing the beneficial effects rather than the placebo effect alone.

During treatment both groups rated the severity of their symptoms (abdominal pain, bloating and bowel habit disturbance) on a daily basis and recorded their general feelings of well-being on a numerical scale. When these scores were compared for the two groups on completion of treatment the differences between them were impressive: the hypnotherapy group showed a dramatic improvement on all measures whereas the control group showed only a minor improvement. During a further study in 1987, Whorwell's original patients were followed up after a period of eighteen months. All patients had remained well, although two had needed a top-up session of hypnotherapy.

The poor response of the control group was rather surprising; many other studies have reported the value of psychotherapy in the treatment of IBS, and it may be that the approach used in the control group was more of a general discussion rather than structured psychotherapy. Nevertheless, although a more structured approach might have reduced the differences between the two groups, this does not detract from the clinical effectiveness of hypnotherapy in IBS. Dr Whorwell's study was the birth of gut-directed hypnotherapy, a technique which is becoming more and more widely accepted.

It has been suggested that the improvement in Whorwell's hypnotherapy patients might have been due to his personality and skill rather than the actual technique, but this has been disputed by other therapists who have produced similar if not almost identical results using the same technique. These studies leave no doubt that it is the technique which is successful rather than the personal attributes of the therapist.

What Actually Happens in Gut-Directed Hypnotherapy?

Before making any attempt to find a therapist it is essential that your condition has been medically investigated and a diagnosis of IBS has been made by a medical practitioner. Your next port of call is to contact a therapist trained in the gut-directed approach (see Appendix).

The Initial Consultation

Having found a therapist you will be asked to attend an initial consultation. This takes about an hour, during which time the therapist will ask you questions about your condition and your general medical history. S/he will listen carefully to all you have to say; it is essential that a good rapport is established in this session. A caring and trusting relationship is a necessary component for successful therapy. S/he will ask detailed questions about your abdominal pain, bloating and bowel habit, and will also ascertain whether you have any problems with your 'upper gut' such as nausea, heartburn, reflux of liquid back into the oesophagus (gullet), etc. S/he will need to know if you have any gynaecological problems or back pain, and whether you feel tired for much of the time. Many of these symptoms are associated with IBS. The therapist may also ask if you have any emotional problems.

After completing the history, the therapist will explain the approach to you. S/he will show you pictures of the inside of your body and explain how the gut functions. Your bowel is a hollow tube surrounded by muscle. This muscle is controlled by the involuntary part of your nervous system, that is, the part which controls your breathing and heart rate – the part you don't usually think about. You will be informed that half of this system psyches you up and half slows you down, and that the system works in a very fine balance. The therapist will go on to explain that the nervous system moves the gut in waves of contraction and relaxation (peristalsis). When you have IBS, the muscles of the gut contract too hard and go into spasm. This causes abdominal pain, bloating and constipation or diarrhoea, or both. S/he will explain that you do have a medical condition (spasm of the bowel can be measured in the laboratory). We do not, however, know what causes the bowel to go into spasm. Many theorists have suggested it may be caused by stress, and although we know that stress has a detrimental effect on the bowel it seems likely that the anxiety and depression reported by many IBS sufferers is secondary to the disorder. Conventional medical treatment often fails, and you may have been told 'There is nothing wrong with you,' 'Learn to live with it,' etc. This approach can only add to your burden. Your debilitating symptoms persist and are at variance with the assertion that nothing is wrong, leaving you in a conflict situation. Because of the effect of emotion on the bowel, this can make your symptoms worse, and you become trapped in a vicious circle where physical symptoms and anxiety reinforce each other.

All this will be discussed in your initial consultation. The therapist will go on to explain that hypnosis itself can help to break this vicious circle and replace it with a healing circle of calmness, relaxation and confidence (CRC). If you are relaxed, it is impossible to be anxious. S/he will then explain what hypnosis is and with the help of a diagram will explain the concept of the conscious and unconscious mind. S/he will explain that we store information in the unconscious part of the mind, and that while most of this information is 'forgotten', these stored events affect the way we think, feel, behave and react. S/he will go on to explain what therapists call the 'critical factor', present in the conscious part of the mind (the part we think with). The critical factor protects us from information which we would prefer not to think about leaking out of the unconscious part of the mind. We do not believe there is a critical component in the unconscious mind, so if we can put positive suggestions in there, they will in turn change the way we think, feel, behave and react.

Hypnosis enables you to relax sufficiently to bypass the critical factor and make this possible.

How the Therapy is Conducted

The therapist then explains that two sessions of CRC therapy backed up by a daily relaxation tape are necessary to prepare your mind for symptom removal. You may have had IBS for many years, and your bowel will have formed a bad habit which will take time to break. After these two sessions s/he will commence gut-directed hypnotherapy. Gut-directed hypno-therapy uses a 'direct suggestion' approach: that is, sugges-tions related to symptom removal are directed into the uncon-scious mind. You will not be required to talk while in hypnosis or to release any uncomfortable emotions. Following induc-tion of hypnosis, ego-strengthening suggestions will be made. Ego-strengthening is a learning process consisting of repetitive suggestions designed to reprogramme your mind into positive thought. When these positive suggestions are repeated time and time again at each session you attend, they become firmly rooted in your unconscious mind and you will gradually notice yourself improving at a psychological level as your thoughts become more positive, confident and optimistic. This is a similar procedure to CRC therapy, but it is more directive and is designed to increase your determination to get well.

Following the ego-strengthener you will be asked to place your hands on your abdomen and generate a sense of warmth and comfort in this area. This is a simple procedure in hypnosis. A sequence of suggestions relating to relaxation of the spasm in your bowel and personal control over gut function will then follow. (Some therapists prefer to use ego-strengthening suggestions after the gut-directed suggestions.) If you have the ability to visualize (make pictures in your mind), the therapist will ask you to visualize a river flowing evenly and comfortably, with no delays or hold-ups, no rushing or hurry. S/he will then ask you to picture the movement through your bowel in the same way. If you are unable to visualize, this option is merely left out of therapy.

How Long Does It Take?

Gut-directed suggestions will be repeated for a further six weekly sessions and you will be expected to play a gut-directed hypnosis tape every day in between treatments. You should by this time be feeling a great deal better, and the next two sessions will be a fortnight apart. If you remain well you will continue with your tape, but have no further sessions for a further four weeks. You will then have a final session before discharge. Once you have this degree of control, you have the wherewithal to control your condition for the rest of your life. There will be times when you have the occasional flare-up (gut-directed hypnotherapy cannot cure IBS), but in most people this is quickly overcome by playing the tape. Booster sessions are offered but are very rarely needed.

The full treatment package will be explained in the initial consultation, and the therapist will tell you that this approach has a very high success rate (eight out of ten patients readily admit to feeling 80 per cent better after a course of treatment) but that the successful outcome depends on you. You need you to be absolutely determined to learn to relax the spasm in your bowel and overcome your symptoms. Often during therapy you will begin to recover and then have a relapse. This is actually good news, because it gives the therapist the opportunity to help you to increase your personal control and determination to get well. Once you have overcome that 'blip' you usually improve steadily; and, more importantly, you will lose your fear of relapses which itself helps to prevent further relapses. Once you have the ability to control any recurrence of abnormal spasm in the bowel the condition is no longer a problem. All in all you will need twelve sessions after the initial consultation for a successful outcome.

Brian

Brian was a 55-year-old IBS sufferer. He had the classic triad of symptoms of pain, bloating and disordered bowel habit and felt tired for much of the time. He suffered from severe diarrhoea, passing up to twelve loose stools per day.

His life had become dominated by his bowel movements. Venturing away from his daily routine was a misery. A day out required careful planning with regard to the whereabouts of public toilets and even a visit to his local town was problematic. Brian's professional background was in science and he wondered how anything as 'airy-fairy' as hypnosis could possibly help him. However, he had a very open mind and was prepared to put his doubts to one side to make the effort needed for successful therapy. Gut-directed hypnotherapy was commenced and he began to improve after four sessions. This improvement was steady apart from a slight 'blip' on all three symptoms halfway through treatment. This was quickly overcome and improvement continued. Brian was discharged after eleven sessions feeling a new man. His energy had returned with all symptoms of IBS eliminated. Follow-up at two years revealed that Brian had remained well. He leads a full life and his bowels are 'not even given a thought'. As he put it: 'Choosing my words deliberately and carefully, gut-directed hypnotherapy literally changed my life.'

Brenda

Brenda was a 32-year-old professional woman. She had classical IBS with alternating constipation and diarrhoea. She had several emotional problems associated with the embarrassment of bloating in public and urgent need of the toilet. Thirteen sessions of gut-directed hypnotherapy coupled with counselling eliminated severe pain, bloating and bowel habit disturbance. On completion of treatment she described herself as 100 per cent well. Follow-up at four years revealed that the benefits have persisted: she has had no flare-ups at all in that time. The latter is welcome but unusual news – most patients have the occasional flare-up from time to time, but they are quickly overcome by using the tape. Brenda has not used her tape since she weaned herself off it after completion of treatment. Brenda concludes by saying: 'When all else had failed, hpnotherapy worked, but I wish it had been suggested as an option sooner.'

Hypnotherapy and Upper Gut Problems

If you have upper gut problems – nausea, heartburn, indigestion, reflux of stomach contents back into the gullet – the therapist will explain that your stomach is either secreting too much gastric acid (a clear fluid secreted by the glands of the stomach to assist digestion) or not emptying as it should. It is a relatively simple procedure to reduce gastric acid secretion or speed up the emptying of the stomach in hypnosis. Your therapist will ask you to place a hand on your stomach; s/he will then make a sequence of suggestions to reduce your gastric acid secretion and/or speed up your gastric motility (movement). Again, this procedure is enhanced by visual imagery if you have this ability. The therapist will include a post-hypnotic suggestion enabling you to control your gastric acid at any time simply by placing your hand in the same position and repeating a trigger word. As your gastric acid becomes normalized, your stomach can contract and empty properly, leaving you free from symptoms. Using this technique, control can be achieved in very few sessions. As with Dr Whorwell's experiments, scientific research has shown that relaxation under hypnosis can result in a significant reduction of gastric acid secretion and gastric motility as compared to a conventional form of relaxation.

Jenny

Jenny is a 48-year-old manager. She has suffered from IBS, with constipation her predominant symptom, since a hysterectomy. She had the classic triad of symptoms, but described her abdominal discomfort as soreness rather than pain. She also suffered from severe heartburn. Gut-directed hypnotherapy was commenced, but Jenny proved to be a poor hypnotic subject and felt that there was 'nothing happening to her'. Nevertheless, despite her misgivings she began to improve after the fourth session. Her heartburn was addressed at the fifth session with the gastric emptying technique described above. This was recorded on tape for her personal use and, as Jenny put it: 'I was astonished; my heartburn, which had been continual for two days, just went!' Both techniques were continued simultaneously for a further five sessions, after which Jenny was discharged, symptom-free. She has the odd 'blip' from time to time which she overcomes herself by using her tape. Jenny states: 'If I hadn't been there, I wouldn't have believed it possible.'

What Alternatives Are There to Gut-Directed Hypnotherapy?

An experienced therapist can usually deduce from disclosures in the initial consultation whether gut-directed hypnotherapy will be sufficient to control your symptoms. Some sufferers may need psychotherapy and/or analytical hypnotherapy before gut-directed hypnotherapy can be successful. Most of us have had traumatic experiences in our lives which can be deeply embedded within the mind. Therapists refer to this process as suppression or repression. These buried events can sometimes have a distorting affect on reality, resulting in unwanted psychological and/or physical symptoms. Working with an altered state of awareness, repressed emotions which are having a harmful effect can be accessed and eliminated. Clients can draw on their imaginative resources and be open to suggestions which encourage more helpful and realistic attitudes. After 'spring cleaning' the mind, the client then has more room to accept gut-directed suggestions, and treatment is usually effective.

This process is known as a psychodynamic approach. If this approach is adopted you will be encouraged to talk through presenting emotional problems. There is a wealth of psychotherapeutic techniques to draw on, and each therapist tends to specialize in one or more areas. The aim, however, is the same in all: to uncover buried traumatic events that are having an adverse effect on your health. When you have gained insight into and understanding of your problems, you can be taught how to deal with them in more constructive ways.

You may decide to undergo hypnotic regression. This is an analytical form of hypnotherapy designed to 'regress' you – take you back – to earlier upsetting events in your life which you have buried and forgotten about. Regression can be carried out in a number of ways. The therapist may establish a diagnostic scan. After fully explaining what s/he is going to do, s/he will then establish an ideo motor response; (IMR). This means s/he will ask your unconscious mind to lift, say, one of your fingers; this happens without any conscious effort on your part. S/he will then count down from your present age down to the first year of your life, suggesting that your finger will lift at each year in which there has been an event or influence which is pertinent to your problem. Establishing the ages that need to be addressed usually takes up one session. In the next session the therapist will start at the top of the list, the age closest to your present age, and while you are in hypnosis s/he will ask your unconscious mind to take you back to that age. You will relive, recall and refeel those events or influences and at the same time your finger will lift to let the therapist know what is going on.

Most people talk through what is happening to them in regression, and this will be appropriately and sympathetically dealt with. This process is known as abreaction or catharsis. When the abreaction is worked through, the therapist will help you to return to the present, and s/he will probably give you some CRC therapy before bringing you out of hypnosis because you are likely to be very tired. You will then have the opportunity to discuss your experience and learn new ways to deal with whatever has come up. This process may sound daunting, but your unconscious mind will protect you and will only allow you to release what it is safe for you to release at that particular time. You will also have formed a trusting relationship with your therapist, who will have had personal experience of regression during training and as a result will be understanding and empathic. Most therapists feel privileged to be allowed to share your emotional problems, and you can be assured that ethical therapists operate within strict confidentiality. The above procedure is repeated session by session until the IMR signals 'clear'. This process in effect clears out the mind, leaving you feeling a great deal better.

Other therapists may use a 'free float' regression. They too will establish an initial scan to get an overall picture, but then, rather than starting at the top and working down, they will use techniques to take you back to whatever event your unconscious mind is willing to deal with at that particular moment. Alternatively, some therapists may use regression to take you straight to the root of whatever is your particular problem. Each practitioner will use his/her discretion as to which is the best approach for you, and the end result is usually the same. Nevertheless, after regression some patients will still have symptoms of IBS, which will then need to be addressed using gut-directed hypnotherapy.

How Can I be Sure that a Therapist is Properly Trained?

If you are going for a psychodynamic approach it is essential that your therapist is qualified in psychotherapy as well as in hypnotherapy. Physicians practising gut-directed hypnotherapy in the National Health Service (NHS) are usually competent in managing the hypnotic state. If it becomes obvious that psychotherapy is necessary and they are not trained in this discipline, they have the facility to draw on hospital psychologists and psychiatrists. In the private sector, however, you need to be able to check that the therapist is properly trained. A competent psychotherapist/hypnotherapist is trained in a number of psychotherapeutic disciplines, which is a lengthy procedure. Thorough training in all aspects of hypnotherapy is also essential. Anyone can learn to induce hypnosis, but management of the hypnotic state is a different business altogether, and the study of applied psychology is just as important as thorough knowledge of hypnotherapy itself. Personal experience of therapy is also desirable and this is an essential part of training. During training students will have undertaken a comprehensive programme of study as well as taking practical and written examinations of a high standard.

An adequately trained therapist will hold a diploma in hypnosis and psychotherapy from a reputable college and will have documentary evidence to this effect. Therapists will belong to an approved association of psychotherapists, which will require them to keep up to date with new developments in the field and to follow a strict code of professional ethics. Such associations also have a disciplinary procedure to deal with any complaints.

The Register of Approved Gastrointestinal Psychotherapists and Hypnotherapists (see Appendix) was formed in 1993 to provide hypnotherapy and psychotherapy to sufferers from gut disorders, both in the private sector and within the NHS. The Register is a properly constituted body with a strict ethical code. You can be sure that all members are professionally trained by a reputable college in both psychotherapy and hypnotherapy before being trained in the gut-directed approach. The Register's constitution requires members to have formal continuing supervision after completing their diploma, and Register members are also required to have additional supervision in the gut-directed approach.

What Happens if I Have Gut-Directed Hypnotherapy and Fail to Improve?

This will become apparent after the first few sessions, and both you and your therapist will need to make a choice either to change the approach or to stop the treatment. If there is no change at all in your condition after six to eight sessions you may conclude that gut-directed hypnotherapy is not going to help you. If this is the case, your therapist will probably already have suggested that you might want to look at yourself in more detail and go for the psychodynamic approach. Most people are happy to do this, but if you are not then do not be persuaded into doing anything against your will. It is your life and your condition, and your views are important. On the other hand, there is little point in continuing gut-directed hypnotherapy, and you may want to think about visiting your general practitioner or trying another form of complementary medicine (see chapter 6 for discussion of these types of treatment).

Mary
Mary is a 45-year-old IBS sufferer who came to us for gut-directed hypnotherapy. She suffered the major triad of symptoms plus upper gut problems. Constipation was her most severe symptom: Mary had not had a bowel move-ment without the use of suppositories for the past eighteen years. She works part-time as a secretary and needed to get up early every morning to use the two or three glycerine suppositories necessary to open her bowels. This perform-ance was causing social, domestic and emotional as well as physical problems. Gut-directed hypnotherapy was having little or no effect on her severe abdominal pain, bloating and constipation, although gastric emptying therapy had reduced her nausea and reflux of gastric acid. Mary was convinced that her constipation was caused by unresolved problems in her childhood. She requested hypnotic regres-sion and this coupled with psychotherapy, proved to be an extremely beneficial but also a lengthy procedure, lasting eighteen months. Hypnoanalysis revealed a number of incidents in childhood that she was 'holding on to'. She thus interpreted her constipation as holding on to the past. She had grown up in a restricted environment with little

freedom to do what she wanted to do. Many traumas were overcome, but a major incident involved her wanting to continue her education after school. This she was denied by her father and as a result she had become dependent on other people's approval for her own happiness. 'I wanted to please my father at the expense of myself.' Resolution of this incident was the beginning of natural bowel movements. Gut-directed hypnotherapy was recommenced and her constipation continued to improve for a period of two months, after which she relapsed. By this time her suppository use had been reduced to half a suppository as necessary. On more and more occasions she was able to open her bowels naturally. It was expected that this relapse would be overcome with direct suggestion, but this was not the case. Counselling revealed that Mary was not particularly happy in her job; deep down she wanted to start her own businss, but was afraid to take the plunge because of her past trauma. Having resolved to go ahead, this time for herself rather than to please others, her bowel began to function once more. Mary reports: 'Therapy taught me not to hold back; I can now make my own important decisions.' Mary still uses the occasional half suppositiory. She has many natural bowel movements but these tend to be irregular. She still has occasional abdominal discomfort, but nevertheless she is choosing to live her life the way she wants to live it and as a result her constipation continues to improve. Mary is slowly being weaned off treatment. She is no longer concerned about her condition and describes herself as 99 per cent well.

Personality and Limitations

Without determination to overcome the symptoms of IBS, gut-directed hypnotherapy will almost certainly fail. Your motivation is the key to a successful outcome. If you are unduly depressed, your motivation will be poor and a short course of anti-depressants from your GP may be helpful to lift your mood sufficiently for treatment to be successful.

Almost everyone can be hypnotized if they want to be. Some people are unable to relax sufficiently because they have a psychological block: that is, they resist deep relaxation for fear of uncomfortable feelings leaking out of the unconscious mind into the conscious. This type of problem would almost certainly need a more psychodynamic approach. Others do not want to be hypnotized for various reasons, including fear of 'mind domination', usually derived from the misconceptions of the stage hypnotist. This can usually be overcome by a sensitive explanation in a trusting, therapeutic relationship. Some patients are afraid that they will not be able to enter the hypnotic state; this also can usually be overcome. Hypnosis is a learned ability and if you want, expect and allow it to happen you will gradually, session by session, drift deeper and deeper into relaxation.

Some patients feel they have not been hypnotized; these are usually in what we call a light trance. Depth is unimportant to a successful outcome (see the case study of Jenny above), but the difficulty is convincing you of this. If you feel nothing has happened you are unlikely to believe that gut-directed hypnotherapy can help you. However, as your symptoms reduce you will become more confident. Light-trance patients sometimes need one or two extra sessions simply to alter their belief that nothing is happening.

The effects of the direct suggestion approach can be influenced by age: we expect less striking improvement in the elderly than in younger or middle-aged sufferers. Nevertheless, I have successfully treated an 88-year-old gentleman. Again, if the elderly are motivated to change direct suggestion is beneficial. Older people can also benefit from gut-directed hypnotherapy combined with general counselling.

A further limitation is a long history of psychological problems; however, this only limits the gut-directed approach. If you belong to this category and are willing to address your emotional problems then a psychodynamic approach followed by gut-directed hypnotherapy can bring about enormous improvements in both your psychological and physical health. The response rate from gut-directed hypnotherapy in patients with chronic constipation coupled with eating disorders tends to be poor. If this is your case, and you are motivated to change, your first step should be to seek a therapist who specializes in eating disorders. When this particular problem has been overcome, gut-directed hypnotherapy may be beneficial.

Attitude is always important. It is necessary to accept that you have IBS, and that this is unlikely to go away. However, if you have no symptoms (or very mild symptoms) then the condition is no longer a problem. If you are expecting a miracle cure from hypnotherapy you will almost certainly be disappointed. As previously mentioned, the major triad of symptoms in classical IBS is abdominal pain, abdominal distension (bloating) and disordered bowel habit. If you have the major triad of symptoms, are not overly psychologically disturbed, are determined to overcome your symptoms and have an open mind, you will almost certainly benefit from straightforward gut-directed hypnotherapy. If you have only one or two of the classical symptoms, success from this approach is less certain; however, if you are not a classical case but are prepared to look closely at yourself, a psychodynamic approach is usually successful.

There is still stigma attached to psychotherapy; please don't let this put you off. Everyone has problems and everyone stores incidents in their unconscious mind. It takes courage and commitment to address the problem, but if they can be released and dealt with in a warm and confidential environment you may feel completely different.

Ellen

Ellen is a 58-year-old professional woman. She had been diagnosed as having IBS six years previously. Her only symptom was severe diarrhoea: up to seventeen loose or liquid stools per day. During the initial consultation it became obvious that she had a multitude of emotional problems. It was these that she wished to address. A diagnostic scan confirmed a host of traumatic incidents in her past. Regression was commenced and one by one these painful memories were brought to the surface. Through this process she gained insight into and understanding of her problems, and supportive psychotherapy helped her to resolve many conflicts. She came to the conclusion that her diarrhoea was an expression of running away from these painful memories, and with that understanding the frequency and urgency of bowel action began to reduce. Ellen is a very strongly motivated lady and put a great deal of effort into her treatment. Regression was completed in sixteen weeks, during which time her diarrhoea had reduced to half without addressing the gut. She needed only six sessions of gut-directed hypnotherapy to complete her treatment. At discharge she had only occasional diarrhoea. On completion of treatment Ellen commented: 'It has been said that love changes everything, but hypnotherapy does it better!' Follow-up after one year revealed that she had continued to improve both psychologically and physically. She gives no thought to her bowels at all and is enjoying life.

In general, diarrhoea-predominant IBS sufferers or those with alternating diarrhoea and constipation tend to respond to gut-directed hypnotherapy better than constipation-predominant sufferers. Nevertheless, the direct suggestion approach has helped a great many constipation sufferers, particularly if they have the classic triad of symptoms.

In my experience sufferers from IBS tend to be intelligent, caring people who are motivated to help themselves. It is this type of individual who will respond best to complementary therapies.

Why is Hypnotherapy Beneficial?

Apart from the obvious explanation that hypnosis is a useful tool with which to access repressed material in the psychodynamic approach, how it is effective in straightforward gut-directed therapy remains a mystery. Various ideas have been put forward. It has been suggested that as hypnosis has a beneficial psychological effect, reduction of stress with increased relaxation and coping skills explains the successful outcome. On the other hand, therapists have found that general CRC therapy, although it reduces anxiety, has little effect on the symptoms of IBS. This explanation also implies that stress is the cause of the condition. An alternative explanation is that hypnosis affects the actual functions of the gut. Dr Whorwell pointed out that the gut and brain share the same nerves and hormones. If emotional and gastrointestinal symptoms are related then physiological changes may be induced by a 'central mechanism' operating at brain level. A study by Whorwell and his colleagues in 1992 looked at the effects of hypnotically induced emotion on the bowel; their results suggested that certain emotions have a striking effect on the bowel of IBS sufferers, and their observation that the induction of hypnosis reduced colonic activity goes some way towards explaining the beneficial effects of gut-directed hypnotherapy in IBS. A further study suggests that improvement in IBS patients after hypnotherapy may be partly due to changes in visceral sensitivity (sensitivity of the abdominal organs). It may also interest readers to know that gut-directed hypnotherapy is clinically effective in cases of inflammatory bowel disease, gastric ulcers and oesophageal problems.

In the absence of more specific facts we can only assume that gut-directed hypnotherapy operates by a variety of mechanisms in IBS patients at both a physiological and a psychological level. Undoubtedly, however, for the vast majority of IBS sufferers, hypnotherapy works either by direct suggestion or as a tool to 'spring clean' the mind.

Availability and Cost

Gut-directed hypnotherapy is available in several NHS hospitals. However, lengthy waiting lists are a problem. It is certainly worth asking your GP if this treatment is available in your local hospital, and asking him/her to refer you. An increasing number of GPs are subscribing to this treatment within their NHS budget, although they tend to treat only their own patients. (See Appendix for physicians practising within the NHS.) The practicalities of obtaining treatment in the NHS are not always straightforward. Once a diagnosis of IBS has been made, you are unlikely to be offered hypnotherapy. Medical treatment together with a sympathetic explanation of your problems will be effective for some people; however, many more are left with a distressing condition that affects them not only physically but socially and emotionally as well. If these people were offered hypnotherapy sooner rather than later, they would probably be spared unnecessary suffering. Apart from this, in the long term there should be a substantial saving to the NHS. It has been argued that it is costly to fund hypnotherapists, which is why gut-directed hypnosis is used only as a last resort: on the other hand, one patient cited above (Ellen) cost £598.44 a year in drugs alone, and had been treated thus for over five years. After hypnotherapy plus a follow-up period of twelve months she was costing the NHS £55.12 per annum, a cost which reflects medication for an additional medical problem: all IBS medication has been discontinued.

We must also consider cost to the state. A number of patients are so debilitated by this condition that they are receiving incapacity benefit. After treatment the majority of patients are able to relinquish their need of benefit and return to work.

Gut-directed hypnotherapy and psychodynamic therapy are available nationally in the private sector through the Register of Approved Gastrointestinal Psychotherapists and Hypnotherapists (see Appendix). Practitioners charge according to their overheads and it is worth shopping around for the right therapist to meet your needs and your pocket.

In the discussion of hypnotherapy in this chapter I hope to have dispelled some of the misconceptions created by stage hypnotists and the media. I have described medical hypnosis as an altered state of consciousness, a pleasant state of relaxation which allows positive suggestions to enter the unconscious part of the mind. I have outlined relevant research and given a detailed account of what to expect in both gut-directed hypnotherapy and analytical hypno-therapy, using illustrative case studies. I have described the limitations of treatment and discussed speculative sugges-tions as to how gut-directed hypnotherapy may operate. The short answer to this question is that we do not know: nevertheless, gut-directed hypnotherapy is extremely effec-tive for the majority of IBS sufferers and the alternative psychodynamic approach is available for those who need it. It remains only to say: 'Having now heard of hypnosis, are you prepared to have a go?'

6

Complementary Alternatives: Treating IBS by Complementary Medicine

Susan Backhouse *

Since the 1980s there has been a surge of interest in 'alternative' or 'complementary' medicine. These terms suggest almost a sideline to traditional western medicine, but in fact many of the various therapies have been successfully healing people for thousands of years. Certain sectors of the medical establishment have often failed to take these disciplines seriously because, it is claimed, there have been few scientific studies to test their efficacy (although more are being undertaken as mainstream interest increases). The practitioners of complementary medicine, however, respond that their results and methods of working are not testable within the framework of conventional medical research. In addition, many will say that they have stood the test of time. An important factor to take into account is that unlike a trial of a new drug, research into complementary medicine does not profit big business concerns; and medical history, in the USA particularly, has been significantly influenced by the financial support of certain training establishments by the pharmaceutical industry. This has meant that since the beginning of the century, mainstream western medicine has become more and more drug-based. Medical training centres

* The author would like to thank Barry Alexander, Kate Burford, Kris Burroughs, Peter Conway-Grim, Dr I. P. Drysdale, Christine Evans, Victor Foster, Nerissa Kisdom, Penny Nunn and Dr Christine Page for their help in preparing this chapter.

which emphasized a more holistic idea of healing were not financed to the same extent and so were more likely to flounder.

Although often thought of as the father of western medicine, the Greek Hippocrates had ideas about health that were very much in tune with those of complementary practitioners. He firmly believed that treatment of a specific complaint should be carried out only as part of the treatment of the whole person; and he stressed the importance of diet to a person's health as well as their habits and the environment in which they lived.

What is Complementary Medicine?

Complementary or holistic medicine, is based on the idea that the physical, emotional and spiritual aspects of a person make up an integrated whole. Each individual is also connected to their family, their environment and the world around them. Thus a practitioner will look at, and attempt to treat, the whole person, rather than particular symptoms or a specific disease. This means that one person with certain symptoms may be given different treatment from another person showing the same symptoms.

A holistic approach is one that sees ill-health as a sign that the body, mind, spirit and emotions are out of balance with each other. It acknowledges the body's great power to heal itself, although therapies may be used to stimulate this power. Holistic medicine does not try to attack a diseased part but aims to support the entire person and guide them in health.

Complementary medicine is different from orthodox western medicine in that the emphasis is on you taking responsibility for your own health and well-being. It is inadvisable to look upon your practitioner, as some people look upon their doctors, as someone to whom you can hand over responsibility for your health. The complementary practitioner should be seen as a facilitator, someone who can support and encourage you, as well as stimulate your body's own unique ability to heal itself.

Choosing a Therapist

Because of the recent increase in interest, there are now many different therapies available to choose from especially if you live in a city. However, the vast majority of them are costly (usually from £20 upwards for an initial session and £15 upwards for treatments thereafter). A few therapies are available on the NHS, and maybe, in time, that will become more common; also, you may be able to attend a training college for a reduced fee. For more information on these colleges, and on NHS availability, contact the umbrella group for the therapy you are interested in (see Appendix). Occasionally, in some areas of the country, complementary practitioners will be part of a local LETS barter scheme (Local Economic Trading Schemes – ask in your library or Citizen's Advice Bureau if there is one near you). But for most people, at the present time, going to a complementary practitioner means parting with a significant sum of money if you want to give it enough of a chance to work. Therefore it is important that you choose your therapist carefully. The following guidelines will help you.

- As the law stands at present, anyone can use the title 'acupuncturist', for instance, whether or not they are adequately trained. To safeguard yourself, contact the umbrella group for the therapy in which you are interested. You will then be able to find out what training those on their register will have had to undertake. You will also be able to enquire about their code of ethics and complaints procedure. They will let you have a list of practitioners in your area.
- Find out about the therapy you are interested in before approaching a particular therapist. Take responsibility for knowing about your own treatment.

- When you make contact with a therapist, ask them how long they have been qualified and whether they are a member of a recognized representative organisation.
- Ask them if the therapy is available on the NHS. If not, ask them how much they charge and whether they operate a sliding scale, if this is relevant to you.
- Ask them if they have had many patients with IBS, and what their success rate with this condition is like.
- Ask them for how long they expect you will need treatment. Although this will only be a guide, and they may be reluctant to pin themselves down, it could give you some idea as to how much the whole course is going to cost you. Treatments for conditions such as IBS often go on for a year or more.
- You may wish to ask them for the name of one of their clients whom you could contact for a reference.
- Ask them if patient records are confidential.
- Ask what insurance cover the practitioner has.

In the following sections the most popular complementary therapies available in this country, and some of the more unusual ones, are discussed in more detail, with particular reference to their use in treating IBS.

Chinese Medicine

Chinese medicine has very ancient beginnings. Over 4,000 years ago a book was written by Huang Ti, the Yellow Emperor, which has much similarity with modern thought on preventative medicine. It states that ailments must be cured before they arise, by proper diet, rest and work, and by keeping the mind and heart calm. This book, the *Nei Ching*, described the circulation of the blood through the body, which was not discovered by the western world until the sixteenth century AD. Anaesthetics were administered by Chinese surgeons as far back as the third century BC, and the catheter, which was 'invented' by western medicine in

1885, was described in a medical book in the seventh century BC. The concept of stress-induced illnesses, thought by some to be a relatively modern idea, was also known to Chinese healers thousands of years ago.

Central to Chinese medicine is the idea that our health depends on the balance of the body's motivating energy or *chi* (pronounced 'chee). *Chi* flows throughout the body but is concentrated in meridians, or channels, underneath the skin. The meridians are connected to the body's organs and functions. *Chi* has two opposite qualities – yin and yang – and the purpose of treatment is to restore the balance between the two. Yang energy represents maleness, light, heat, dryness, contraction, strength, activity, sun, spring, summer; yin is characterized by femaleness, receptivity, tranquillity, darkness, coldness, moisture, swelling, weakness, passivity, earth, autumn and winter. Although yin and yang are opposites, they are not hostile to one another. Each needs the other; without one, the other could not exist. Yang is not superior to yin, nor is yin superior to yang. Contrast this concept with traditional western thinking where masculinity is superior to femininity, objective is better than subjective, quantity is better than quality, body better than mind, activity better than passivity. Chinese medicine teaches that the whole order of the universe results from the perfect balance between the two forces of yin and yang, and that similarly our health depends on this crucial balance within our bodies.

Yin and yang are represented, for example, by the dilation and contraction of the heart; the exhalation and inhalation of the lungs; and the functions of the parasympathetic and sympathetic nervous systems. According to the Chinese, all diseases are the result of an imbalance between yin and yang. In the body, too much yang manifests itself as acute pain, inflammation, spasms, headache, high blood pressure, irritability and excitation. Too much yin might appear as dull aches, chilliness, fluid retention and discharges and is characterized by weakness, exhaustion and debility. By restoring the balance of the energy system, Chinese medicine aims to stimulate the body's own healing powers.

Modern western medicine is coming to the same conclusions in some respects. For instance, many western physicians believe that if the sympathetic and parasympathetic nervous systems are not in harmony with each other, illness will surely follow. Science tells us that a harmonious functioning of the nervous systems and a well-balanced disposition is essential in order to avoid some of the stress-induced diseases which are so rampant today – high blood pressure, heart trouble, stomach ulcers, headaches, insomnia, etc.

Chinese medicine teaches that the stomach and spleen (pancreas) are the 'mothers' of the bowel. The idea is that if the 'mother' is tired and therefore deficient she cannot properly nourish the 'child', in this case, the colon. A practitioner of Chinese medicine would aim to strengthen these organs together with the bowel for anyone suffering from a bowel disorder.

Chinese medicine also sees the emotions of grief, melancholy and sadness as inherent to colon energy or *chi*. Not only is the colon affected adversely by these emotions from without but it can itself give rise to these emotions, which are believed to exacerbate IBS. It might be interpreted that an IBS sufferer is holding on to some sort of grief, or harbouring a sense of loss. There may be deep disappointment about oneself, one's own life, the hopes and dreams one had, and this will affect the bowel quite profoundly. Chinese lore teaches that it is essential to give up these emotions that one might be holding to give the bowel a good chance of recovery.

Acupuncture

Acupuncture is an ancient medical system, dating back over 2,000 years. The word itself is a western word meaning 'needle piercing', but the Chinese term is *chen chiu*, which means 'needle moxa'. Moxa is a dried herb which is sometimes burned on the skin or on the end of the needles to create a gentle heat which facilitates the treatment.

The ideas of having needles stuck in your body has been alien to many westerners until recently. It sounds as if it would be very painful. However, the needles used in acupuncture are so fine that when they are inserted it is usual to feel nothing more than a slight tingle.

For those people who are afraid of needles, or for children, the acupuncture points of the body can be massaged or pressure can be applied with a probe. Modern technology has seen the arrival of electro-acupuncture and laser treatments in which the acupuncture points are stimulated by a low-frequency electrical current, applied with a probe or with finely tuned laser beams.

It has been discovered that the stimulation of acupuncture points induces the release by the brain of morphine-like substances called 'endorphins', which have pain-relieving properties; acupuncture is used extensively for pain relief, and has been used as an alternative to anaesthetic in many surgical operations.

The theory behind acupuncture has been developed through the ages and is based on the idea that the meridians, along which flows the life energy, or *chi*, are connected to the body's organs and functions, and along these meridians are found the points that the acupuncturist manipulates in order to regulate the flow of energy and restore health. Although there doesn't seem to be a definite anatomical structure to the points, they can be detected electronically.

An acupuncturist will attempt diagnosis by careful and thorough questioning and observation. You will be asked about past illnesses, details of the current problem, your general energy level, and family traits and tendencies. Your practitioner will attempt to assess the functioning of all your body's systems, and your face and body features will be carefully observed. You will be asked about your response to changes in the weather, your taste preferences, your feelings and phobias. On each visit your pulse will be felt and your tongue will be inspected. The acupuncturist will aim to build up a full picture of you so that your current problem can be seen in perspective.

With the rise of AIDS there has been some concern about the safety and hygiene aspects of acupuncture treatment. The British Acupuncture Association and Register say their members have to use needle sterilization techniques approved by the Department of Health, which are considered to be completely effective against hepatitis and AIDS. Many practitioners use disposable needles.

Acupuncturists will say that they treat the person, not the disease, so a question such as 'Can acupuncture cure IBS?' can only be asked as 'Can this person be cured of their IBS using acupuncture?', and can only be answered after the practitioner has examined the patient; but it is said that acupuncture can have an effect on almost any illness so long as the degenerative process in the tissues of the body is not too extensive. Many practitioners will work in cooperation with other therapists if it is deemed to be useful in particular cases.

One practitioner believes that acupuncture is very effective in IBS cases where the link with stress is strong. He says that in his experience, those patients whose stress is relieved by the treatment get much better, while those whose stress stays much the same don't improve. As it is believed that acupuncture can be particularly helpful in alleviating stress, if you feel this is a major factor in your IBS it may be worth a try. The same practitioner says that he would normally expect some change after three or four treatments, with significant improvement after ten. If there is no result after ten sessions, he advises trying something else.

It is worth noting that as some acupuncture points are not suitable for use on pregnant women, it is important to tell your practitioner if you are. This advice would apply for any therapy.

Lizzie has been receiving acupuncture for a year. She's 40 years old and has had IBS for five years. She has been happy with the way her acupuncturist has treated her and has found him to be very sympathetic. He has attempted to get a picture of her as a whole person and to try and understand what the reasons might be behind her symptoms.

However, she says:

> 'I feel that the sessions don't really help as much as I might have hoped. I usually feel better for a day or two after each session but the symptoms get worse again. Sometimes I feel that the symptoms increase again when I am nervous or tense. Occasionally I get panic attacks when I am alone and my insides go crazy. I feel a bit silly admitting this as outwardly I appear to be confident. I have scarcely mentioned this to the practitioner. I pay £22 per acupuncture session and wonder whether I am wasting money but continue to go.'

As well as the acupuncture treatment, Lizzie was given dietary advice – a balanced wholefood diet avoiding coffee, too much wheat and alcohol.

Gillian, who suffers from chronic constipation, first tried acupuncture twenty years ago. She attended the sessions weekly for some months. She found it very beneficial and achieved a better bowel function. However, when she stopped the treatment the constipation returned.

She later saw another acupuncturist but this time experienced no benefit and the practitioner advised her not to continue the treatment, which Gillian felt was honest of her.

A third time, Gillian found the needles very painful and was unable to continue the acupuncture because the discomfort was causing a lot of tension. Interestingly enough, a non-IBS-related stomach problem cleared up soon after.

Caroline is aged 43 and had had IBS for over ten years. She originally went to her acupuncturist for neck and arm pain; this disappeared after five treatments and her IBS also greatly improved.

Chinese Herbalism

Richard Lucas, in his book *The Secrets of the Chinese Herbalists*, says that these healers do not claim to cure anything:

rather, they simply work to support and assist nature in its endeavour to heal the ailing organism. The herbalists of China believe that non-poisonous plant medicines supply to the body the appropriate constituents it lacks, in a way similar to natural foods.

Chinese herbalists use many herbs for bowel disorders, including yellow dock (normalizer and regulator of bowel function), blackberry root (astringent, with a strengthening effect when used as a remedy for diarrhoea), slippery elm (soothing, mucilaginous, assures easy passage during bowel movements, absorbs foul gases in the body) and garlic (used as a remedy for diarrhoea and other intestinal disturbances, anti-bacterial).

Shiatsu

Japanese shiatsu is based on the meridian energy system as applied in traditional Chinese medicine. Instead of needles, the Shiatsu therapist uses touch to rebalance the energy or *chi* at relevant points along the meridians – or anywhere on the person which is felt to be either in excess of, or deficient in, energy. The aim is to tone and strengthen the particular functions of the organs within the body, as well as give a feeling of well-being and deep relaxation. The practitioner applies pressure to the body using thumbs, hands, elbows, knees or feet. Stretching and structural adjustments may also be used. The recipient is clothed and lies or sits on a futon mattress on the floor.

Kris Burroughs explains her view of IBS as a shiatsu therapist:

'The large intestine is closely associated with the lung and also the skin in Chinese medicine. These form an immediate interface with the external environment and a means of cleansing the body from waste and toxins. IBS can be associated with retaining the breath in the chest and an inability to let go, to exhale the carbon dioxide-loaded breath. This can be likened to a state of constipation and retention of the faeces in the colon.

'I would work with the breath, as a means both of cleansing and of releasing physical and emotional holding patterns. Often IBS sufferers feel a need to control themselves and memories of trauma over childhood toilet training (control or lack of control of their anal sphincter) may surface. Perhaps that their shit, or how or where they shit, wasn't OK. This may have led to over-control or a disownership of that part of themselves. There may be alternating patterns of withdrawing into themselves for security (constipation) and moving out into the world in a more assertive or retaliating way (diarrhoea).

'Problems with the colon are often related to the spleen, the "mother" of the colon in Chinese medicine. This is associated with nourishment, security and a sense of inner trust of the self. If there has been insufficient mothering and mixed messages about both physical and emotional feeding, this will necessarily affect the kind of digestion, absorption and retention of food and how we feel about our products of digestion.'

She goes on to describe how she treats a client:

'A session usually begins with palpation of the *hara* [belly] – the central reservoir of our *chi* – and this enables the practitioner to decide which meridians to focus on during the session and is itself a treatment. In fact, the entire shiatsu session can be viewed as both diagnosis and treatment – not only where and how the practitioner touches but what form of verbal communication takes place with the client. This may range from emotional counselling to advice about physical exercise, spiritual practice or diet.'

Many therapists believe that a healthy way of eating is essential for people with IBS. Shiatsu practitioner Barry

Alexander says that slow and thorough chewing of the food is of supreme importance because, he says,

'If animal or vegetable protein hits the bowel incompletely digested in the previous stages of gut absorption, then the caecum section of the colon will be forced to flood that whole area of the colon with white blood cells to neutralize this rotting protein. Because the colon is not designed to deal with undigested protein particles it protects itself in this way, but inefficiently, and the detrimental effect to the colon gives rise to the multitude of pathologies associated with IBS and other related colon problems.'

A shiatsu practitioner may accompany his or her treatment on the large intestine meridian with special techniques incorporated in what is called *hara* (belly) massage. S/he may also recommend the Japanese way of self-massage of the abdomen or *ampuku*, which can be very effective. It is believed to prevent stagnation of blood, fluids and *chi*, which can cause various problems including bowel disorders. An additional technique which the patient may practise for his or herself is to stimulate the acupuncture point Colon 4, which is between the index finger and thumb, above the web, on the fleshy part. This is something that can be done yourself by massaging the point, using your other thumb in an upward direction towards the wrist) and towards the index finger. The point can be massaged on both hands.

Barry Alexander says that treatment for IBS must be consistent if absolute improvement is to be obtained. He believes that in the early days treatment should be at least weekly, maybe for the first eight sessions. After improvement, sessions can be less frequent. Successful shiatsu treatment will stimulate *chi* so that the bowel can be regenerated and healed; full recovery of the bowel may take up to a year, depending on the severity of the problem. He goes on to say:

'It is important to choose a shiatsu practitioner who possesses strong *chi* in him/herself and can project it to where he/she wants it to go. In this way, spectacular results can be achieved. It also matters how the practitioner thinks. If there is no conviction in his/her treatments, the results will not be good.'

And on *chi*:

'*Chi* is that force which accompanies all of life, without which there is none. *Chi* is the very energy and meaning in the message you are reading right now. It is the desire to help. It is the power behind vitality. It is grace in all its meanings, and is the power behind action.'

Denise tried shiatsu for a number of conditions including IBS. She has had IBS for over ten years and had frequent acute abdominal pains which were very difficult to deal with and which were not relieved by anti-spasmodic drugs. She speaks well of the therapist, whom she enjoys going to see and whom she finds very supportive and sympathetic towards her health problems. She reports feeling very relaxed once the treatment is over. Since her first visit some months ago, she has had no pains from IBS.

Homoeopathy

The principles of modern homoeopathy were established in the eighteenth century by a physician, Dr Samuel Hahnemann. He was disillusioned by the medical practices of the time, which so often did more harm than good. He believed that we humans have the ability to heal ourselves and that the physician's task is to discover, and if possible remove, the cause of the trouble, and to stimulate the body's own vital healing force. By experimenting on himself and his supporters he discovered that many substances which caused illness in a healthy person would ease symptoms in someone who was ill; amazingly, he also discovered that the smaller the dose he used, the more effective it was. The homoeopathic remedy is produced by a special method of dilution until very little of the original substance is left. It is then given in tablet, liquid, granule or powder form.

The remedies are given with the intention of removing symptoms by rebalancing energies in the body. In contrast to the approach in conventional western medicine, and as in other complementary therapies, the patient is treated rather than the disease. This means that one person with IBS might be given different remedies from another person suffering from the same condition, even the same symptoms.

The remedies come from many different sources. Homoeopaths use plants; substances like sand, charcoal, salt and pencil lead; drugs like morphine, cocaine and arsenic; but all are diluted in the special manner so that poisons are no longer poisonous, innocuous substances become effective and all have great power for healing – for the right person; for anyone else they would have no effect. Because of the minute doses involved there are no side effects, although as the healing starts symptoms may get worse before getting better. Homoeopathic remedies are safe for babies and children, and for pregnant women.

During the first consultation the practitioner will take a detailed case history of the patient. Homoeopaths have a particular interest in what makes the symptoms worse or better, for example, certain foods, stress, warmth or cold, etc. They will look at the general health of the individual, the aspects of his or her personality which make them unique as well as the particular symptoms being experienced. As the patient's personality is often discussed in some depth, it will inevitably lead to some counselling. Dr Christine Page, a medical doctor and practising homoeopath, believes that all homoeopaths should have some counselling skills or be ready to refer the patient to a specialist.

Dr Page describes what she looks for at the first consultation:

'Having taken a full homoeopathic history, I, personally, also take a history of a daily diet and check that there are no excesses (or deficiencies) in the diet. Foods which are known to make IBS worse include wheat products, tea, citrus fruits and tomatoes. The problem of candida overgrowth would also be assessed, especially if there is a history of recurrent antibiotics. Dietary advice may well be given or referral to a nutritionist.

'In the first consultation I aim to record a set of parameters which relate to the specific illness, general health and the mind. From these I select one remedy from thousands which hopefully matches these parameters as closely as possible. This remedy may be given as a single dose or regular doses, depending on the individual. With homoeopathy, once the symptoms clear you stop the treatment. Even with one powder it is possible to see the cessation of all symptoms for life.'

She goes on to describe the part she believes personality has to play in IBS:

'My own feeling is that IBS is associated with relationship issues when the patient is often uncomplaining and lets things go, rather than speaking out. [He or she] looks for peace rather than conflict. There is often a love/hate relationship especially with family and a need for both closeness and space and yet an inability to ask for either. There is also a strong conscientious energy, trying to do a good job and yet often resenting the neediness of others.'

Dr Julie Allen has been a practising homoeopath for over twenty years and has a high success rate with IBS sufferers. She uses hypnotherapy and psychotherapy with homoeopathy and believes that a large part of the problem with IBS is of a psychological nature. She says that in the majority of patients that she has treated over the years, stress, anxiety and deep-rooted psychological problems have predominated. If the patient is unwilling to change their lifestyle and attitude, she says, they may only obtain temporary relief from either homoeopathic or conventional medicine.

Maria is in her seventies and has suffered from IBS for about thirty-five years. When she was diagnosed as having 'spastic colon' in 1963 her consultant told her she would be on drugs for the rest of her life. She wasn't helped in any way and became dependent on the Libraxin she was prescribed. After a year, she was determined to wean herself off the drug, and did so over the next six months.

What Maria found hardest to deal with was the many days when she felt completely unwell – feverish, constipated, with a feeling of general malaise. The only way of getting over it was to go to bed for two days and to eat just stewed cooking apples and milky rice pudding.

Her practitioner treats her with both acupuncture and homoeopathy. When she first went she was very ill with her symptoms. She was relieved to find that in the practitioner she found for the first time someone who knew what she was talking about and who did not treat her symptoms as of no account, a waste of time.

'She said she had treated other people with this trouble, she could improve the quality of my life, renew my energy, and make me feel much better – she did *not* say she could "cure" me. I began to feel better very soon, and this was lasting, although it was several months before I was feeling really well.'

Maria found that tension in her lower back disappeared, as did a swelling of fluid under her skin that had been there for a year, which was proof to her that the treatment was working. After going every three weeks, she now attends three-monthly sessions for a general booster. She also has a Bach Flower formula to suit her (see page 154) and the practitioner also recommended a slippery elm drink and Quiet Life tablets. At £25 for the first consultation and £15 for each visit thereafter, Maria feels it is expensive but worth every penny:

'I still have some of the symptoms at times, but never so severe, and only very infrequently, after great stress, for instance. I am now much stronger and fitter than I have been for many years. It is such a pleasure to be well after nearly half my life drifting from one ill patch to the next.'

Angie is a 40-year-old nurse and was diagnosed with Irritable Bowel Syndrome some twenty years ago. Her symptoms were relatively mild up until the last three years, when she has suffered with more diarrhoea, abdominal pain, severe nausea, bloating and wind. A year ago she began to see a homoeopath who is also a medical doctor:

'She has helped me to recognize certain patterns and issues in my life with which I wasn't dealing effectively and how this was affecting my physical health. Her treatments helped me feel stronger and more confident – people commented I seemed like a different person – with a resultant decrease in IBS symptoms, but, more importantly, [it gave me] the ability to cope more effectively with them and not go to pieces when they did occur.'

Not everybody speaks of homoeopathy so highly. Gwynneth is a 75-year-old housewife and retired teacher. She has suffered from diarrhoea and nausea for the last two years. She saw a homoeopath for six months, and spent £80, but felt it did not relieve her symptoms. The practitioner suggested she tried the Hay Diet for the diarrhoea, and this was of some help.* However, she stopped the treatment when she began to feel that the remedies he was giving her (primarily for sinusitis) were contributing to her bowel problems.

Treatment may last years, as Maureen found out. She has been seeing a homeopath for four and a half years:

'This may seem like a long time, but one of the first things she told me was that there was no quick cure, just a long-

---

* The theory behind the Hay System is that starches and sugars shouldn't be consumed at the same meal as protein and acid fruits.

standing improvement. During my course of treatment the pills have been changed many times and I still take two pills every other day, or every day if needed.

For the past year I have been 90–95 per cent free from IBS – I won't say cured as I still have little setbacks.'

Because of another health condition Maureen's homoeo-path advised a diet that is very low in fat but contains lots of fruit, vegetables and salads. Previous to her homoeopathic treatment, Maureen says, her diet was very poor because of a recommendation by a hospital consultant to omit any foods she had eaten prior to an IBS attack.

Herbalism

The use of plants for healing goes back, no doubt, as far as we humans do! Archaeological information has shown that Neanderthal people of 60,000 years ago may have had knowledge of medicinal plants. In the beginning, prehistoric men and women probably put most plants into their mouths. Many were innocuous, some were nourishing, some made them ill and a few killed them. Some, they found, relieved symptoms of sickness or pain and a few caused halluci-nations. Those plants in the last two categories became their medicines.

Much of our knowledge of herbalism has been acquired over the ages by trial and error and handed down from one generation to another. It is only really in this century that herbal or 'natural' remedies have *not* been at the forefront of medicine. On more than one occasion in recent years, scientists have developed a drug that is less effective and more toxic than the original herbal remedy. Of course, there are areas in which herbal medicine has remained important, especially in the pockets of surviving aboriginal cultures where modern western medicine has remained relatively unknown and where plants still provide the only medicines.

Medical herbalists disagree profoundly with the orthodox

or 'allopathic' approach of finding, isolating and synthesizing an active ingredient from a plant – for example, aspirin from willow bark, quinine from cinchona bark, digoxin from foxglove, etc. They believe that the active ingredient, when taken out of the context of the whole plant, is incompatible with good health: there are many other elements in the whole plants which have an important part to play in the natural balance. For example, dandelion leaves are a strong diuretic; but it is not necessary to give a potassium supplement with them, as is usually required with a drug diuretic, as they are a rich source of potassium themselves.

Like many other complementary therapies, herbalism aims to stimulate the body's own powers of healing. It does not suppress the symptoms; rather, it assists in the restoration of balance and harmonious functioning of the body. Toxins are encouraged to be discharged, which can often make the patient feel quite unwell for a short time while the cleansing process is taking place. This is important as an underlying toxicity would, herbalists believe, prevent a lasting equilibrium from being established.

Although you can buy herbs and herbal remedies for specific complaints over the counter, qualified herbalists would say that they will treat you as a whole person, rather than a collection of symptoms. A herbal preparation made specifically for you by an experienced practitioner will address the underlying imbalance, rather than simply aim to alleviate the surface symptoms. Herbalist Peter Conway-Grim points out:

> 'The interest in peppermint oil is a good example. Peppermint can be useful in the treatment of IBS, but only in certain circumstances and within certain limits. When treated as mere pills to be popped, herbs will be only occasionally effective. Likewise, the quality of herbs is also important. The chamomile [which has anti-inflammatory, sedative and tissue-healing effects on the gut] used in

commercial teabags is not of medicinal standard and will be unlikely to offer much help.

Another herbalist, Christine Evans, looks at diet and dietary habits in great detail, often with the use of questionnaires, so that she can make recommendations as to how they might be altered to help the healing process. The first consultation includes a detailed investigation of the whole patient. It may take an hour or more and includes an in-depth medical history, abdominal palpation, examination of the irises, skin, tongue, nails and other physical diagnostic features. Christine looks for general signs of the patient's overall condition such as signs of debility, and physical, mental and emotional exhaustion. Blood pressure and pulse are assessed.

She describes how she prescribes with the IBS patient in mind:

'The herbal formulae chosen would be quite individual, being composed of a number of complementary herbs which would not only address the root cause, but [also] strengthen weakened organs and systems within the body. For instance, anti-inflammatory, antispasmodic, demulcent, soothing and cleansing herbs may be given to heal the intestinal wall, along with herbs to tonify or calm the nervous system, provide nourishment and balance specific related organs such as the liver, pancreas, spleen or kidneys. In addition, any nutritional deficiencies that are frequently present are assessed and corrected. This is very important as many patients are severely debilitated which impairs the body's ability to heal. The herbs themselves supply vital nutrients in an easily assimilable form, thus strength and vitality is restored and many other seemingly unrelated symptoms are frequently improved.'

After years of suffering and misery, when she seemed to be getting worse and worse, Patsy decided to get rid of all her drugs and as a last resort to try a local clinic of herbal medicine run by a former nurse and midwife. The herbalist told her she was run down because of the continuous diarrhoea she suffered, and she was put on thirteen different minerals and nutrients straight away. She was advised to go on the Hay Diet and to avoid all processed foods, tea and coffee. Patsy was also put on a three-day fast which, she was told, was a cleansing process to rid her body of all the toxins she had accumulated. She felt quite ill for a day or so, with severe headaches, but was told this was to be expected, like going through 'cold turkey' after giving up drugs. Two years ago, she wrote:

'I stuck it out as I thought anything was worth it to get rid of my IBS. I have slowly got better. For the past three months I have not had diarrhoea at all. My nails and skin have improved and many people tell me I look so much better. Also, my blood pressure has reduced so I have also been able to cut down on the tablets I have been taking for fifteen years for that.

The downside of this is that it has so far cost me £200 which, as a pensioner, has been difficult to find, but it has been worth it.'

One of the clinics run by this herbalist is now able to take patients who have been referred by their GP at reduced fees.

Gillian visited a different herbalist many years ago. After a very thorough medical history was taken, she was prescribed a medicine which was to help a number of problems she had apart from constipation. She consulted the practitioner every four to six weeks and, although the medicines she was prescribed were generally helpful, she didn't sustain any long-term improvement to any of her health problems, including her IBS.

Naturopathy

Naturopathy is a philosophy and therapy which aims, like many other complementary therapies, to stimulate the body to us its own power to heal itself. The philosophy, and some of the methods used in naturopathy, date back to at least 400 BC (although 'modern' naturopathy is about a hundred years old), when Hippocrates stated that only nature heals, providing it is given the opportunity to do so. He also believed in the importance of food as medicine and that disease is an expression of purification.

The philosophy of naturopathy is based on three principles: (1) that the body has the power to heal itself through its own vital force; (2) that disease is the body's way of trying to get rid of anything that is preventing its organs and tissues from functioning properly, whether this is chemical (e.g. an imbalance in the body's chemistry due to dietary deficiency or excess), mechanical (e.g. physcial damage due to poor posture or injury) or psychological (e.g. illness caused by stress and anxiety); (3) that naturopathy looks at the whole person – body, mind and spirit – and sees the patient as a unique individual who might respond and react quite differently to the next person.

According to the General Council of Naturopaths:

> The task of naturopathic practitioners is twofold. First, to educate their patients to take more responsibility for their health and to assist them to understand the fundamental laws of health relating to rest, exercise, nutrition and lifestyle. Second, using natural therapies, to increase the vitality of the individual and to remove any obstructions, chemical, physical or psychological, which may be interfering with the normal functioning and internal harmony of the organs and tissues.

A practitioner might use various therapies to stimulate the healing process, including prescription of a natural diet, which may or may not be specific and controlled, depending on the practitioner and the patient; fasting; structural adjustment such as osteopathy, chiropractic and remedial exercises to rebalance the body; hydrotherapy, which is the use of water in various ways, both internally and externally; advice on a healthy lifestyle – relaxation, exercise, the cultivation of a positive attitude, etc; and education, so that the patient is able to take responsibility for their own health. It isn't unusual for the patient to experience an initial worsening of their symptoms as part of what is called 'the healing crisis'.

Naturopaths aim to help restore their patients to a point where they no longer have a use for treatment and can maintain good health themselves through whole food, fresh air, exercise and positive thinking.

Dr I. P. Drysdale of the British College of Naturopathy and Osteopathy has this to say about treating patients with IBS:

'Practitioners such as ourselves treat individual patients uniquely. However, there are certain basic elements of treatment which are common to most sufferers of IBS. For example, the types of treatment that a naturopathic osteo-path would use are minipulation of viscera [organs of the abdomen], together with dietetic advice and a certain amount of counselling advice, stress being an important input to the IBS syndrome.

'What I think is unique about our particular philosophy is that we combine rational dietetics with counselling and a physical hands-on treatment, and this approaches the patient's situation on at least three levels. As these three are integrated from the practitioner point of view, we feel this is most beneficial to the patient.

'Generally when treating irritable bowel syndrome, it ultimately depends on patient cooperation and willingness to follow the particular lifestyle outline that is given.'

Katie was recommended to a college of naturopathy and osteopathy by her reflexologist. The following is her account of her treatment there.

'The first visit cost £15 for an hour's consultation and treat-ment. Further visits cost £10 for half an hour. They work on the basis of treating the whole person and look at body structure, mental make-up and biochemistry (nutrition).

'On the first visit I discussed my symptoms with a trainee osteopath who was due to qualify at the end of the month. She took details of my medical history, including any previous operations, and asked whether I was taking any medications. I explained the symptoms of IBS and she asked whether I had had any previous treatment.

'She asked me to undress to my underwear and stand in front of her. She checked my posture and felt along my spine, and also felt around my stomach/colon area. She then left the room to discuss her notes and diagnosis with a qualified osteopath. (A fully qualified osteopath will see you if the student is not sure about anything.)

'When she came back into the room, she explained that my colon on the left side was very 'tight' and constricted and this is why the muscle went into spasm. She then explained how she would manipulate various muscles in my stomach and belly area.

'She pressed quite hard along the line of my colon and it was quite sore on the left-hand side. She also worked on an area to the left of my lower back which she told me corresponds with the digestive system. This was very painful. She worked on these areas for about ten minutes.

'At the end of the session, she asked me to complete a diet sheet and to post it back to her. This recorded everything I ate for one week. She also showed me how to massage the colon area myself and said I should do this for a few minutes every day if possible. She said that by doing this I would help to push the contents along and disperse any gas.

'Since I saw her I have had no morning upsets at all. [Previously, Katie had regularly passed frequent loose motions in the morning.] My colon area was quite sore for a few days, as was the area in my lower back where she had been treating me. I have had just one movement most days, although some days I have gone once more after lunch or later on. On these days I feel unwell until I go to the toilet for a second time. I have only had one day when

I went three times in total. I have not used Imodium at all since the first visit.

'On the second visit, my diet was discussed. I was advised to try to cut down, or preferably cut out, sugary drinks and have plain water or fruit juices diluted with water instead. I should have a bowl of salad each day to include two green leafy vegetables. I was also asked to try to eat protein foods separately from carbohydrates. It was suggested that I should change what I have for breakfast as I usually have a cereal such as Rice Krispies which contain a lot of sugar. Unfortunately this discussion took up the whole half-hour appointment and I was disappointed that there was no time for any treatment.

'I have booked a third appointment as the osteopath said that I would probably benefit from three or four more treatments, although this was for [another problem] rather than the IBS. She said that by continuing to massage my colon myself, I could keep the problem under control and altering my diet would help to 'clean up' my system.

'I really do feel that this is the answer to my problems. I just wish that my own doctor had advised me of the benefits of massage to the colon when I first had IBS.'

Reflexology

The principle of reflexology is that there are reflex areas in the feet and hands which correspond to all of the glands, organs and parts of the body and that these can be manipulated by using the thumb and fingers on these areas.

Reflexology has been used for 5,000 years in China, but at the beginning of the century an American called Dr William Fitzgerald claimed to have discovered that there are ten electrical currents running through the body from the top of the head to the toes. All the organs, glands and nervous systems of the body fall within the areas covered by these currents. The theory is that crystalline deposits form around the nerve endings, preventing the electrical currents from earthing through the hands and feet. Pressure on the hands and feet will break up the deposits and allow the currents to 'earth', restoring balance and enabling a smooth flow of energy throughout the body.

It was in the 1930s that Eunice Ingham charted the feet in relation to the corresponding areas of the body. She developed a map of the feet which related to the entire body, all parts being related to specific areas, or reflexes, on the hands and feet. Sensitivity in a particular area on the foot is believed to be a sign that there is congestion or tension in the corresponding part of the body. Pressure and manipulation on that part of the foot sets in motion therapeutic benefits within the body.

Reflexology aims, like many other therapies, to create a balance within the body in order that good health may be achieved or maintained. A consultation will start with the practitioner feeling the feet and noting where the sensitive areas are. A case history may then be taken. The feet will then be massaged and pressure applied, paying particular attention to those areas which indicate crystalline deposits and blocked energy. Most people find the treatment extremely relaxing and soothing, even though some areas of the feet may be quite sensitive. Results may be seen after two or three sessions, but in cases of long-standing disorders progress may take a lot longer.

Nadia is 43 and has had IBS for a year. She was told that it was probably caused by a hysterectomy she had had some months previously. Her symptoms include passing stools about five times in the morning, which is exhausting for her and causes her to feel very low and anxious first thing. She says she finds it difficult not knowing what each day will be like; knowing that some days she can be 100 per cent, but not knowing why, and on other days feel so bad she just wants to stay indoors.

Nadia has been receiving reflexology treatment recently and has been weekly for seven weeks. She pays £14 for an hour. She has found the practitioner very sympathetic, questioning her thoroughly about her general health as well as IBS, listening well and remembering every detail. After six treatments Nadia noticed a great improvement and felt elated; but sadly it only lasted for a week.

She would recommend that other sufferers try reflexology, mainly because she believes anything is worth a shot. She, herself, found it a worrying treatment, however, because:

> 'She kept picking up other points of the body that indicated trouble; in my case it was neck, shoulder, adrenal gland, spleen, urethra and womb – which I haven't got!'

Stephanie saw a practitioner who treated her with aromatherapy and homoeopathy as well as reflexology. Her symptoms consisted of wind, severe constipation, urgent visits to the toilet in the morning and cramping pains, as well as panic, lack of energy and a general feeling of unwellness. She received the treatment weekly for a year. Stephanie was pleased with the practitioner's sympathetic and caring attitude. She wasn't cured by the treatment but, as she says, it was helpful:

> 'The treatment helped to a certain extent by relaxing me, as by that time I was extremely tense and probably at my lowest level. However, the relief was not really beneficial in the long term. I must stress, though, that mentally it helped greatly as, having been told by the medical profession that this was just the way I was and I would have to live with it, I felt so alone and uptight. I was becoming afraid to leave the house. I no longer felt alone and was extremely thankful that someone felt I wasn't a stupid woman who was probably imagining all these symptoms anyway.'

Katie tried five sessions of reflexology for her IBS. She was very happy with the practitioner, who treated her for two hour sessions at the one-hour rate of £15, made various dietary suggestions and discussed her case with other therapists for ideas, but although stiffness in her neck benefited, her IBS did not improve at all.

Rena was sceptical about trying reflexology at first, but her story is a positive one. As she says:

'I am the type of person that shuns various herbs and home remedies but when my IBS was at its peak, I was persuaded to try it. I had a treatment and was violently ill the next day. I had another the following week and can honestly say I felt better. I had two more treatments in five weeks and I now have a treatment every five weeks. My reflexologist has put together a small potion of herbs and liquidized it and if I feel unwell, I rub a little on my stomach at night and by next morning I feel fine. I am pleased to say that apart from the odd bout I have been virtually IBS-free.'

Colonic Irrigation

Colonic irrigation, or colonic hydrotherapy, is a technique which was apparently first recorded in 1500 BC and has been used by various traditional and complementary practitioners since then. Using sterilized equipment, warm, filtered water is gently introduced through the rectum and into the colon. Special massage techniques are used so that the water progressively softens and expels faecal matter and compacted deposits, which are then piped away with the waste water. The idea is that it rids the body of the build-up of toxins in the gut which can otherwise be reabsorbed into the blood, causing, or contributing to, a variety of illnesses.

A session takes about thirty minutes. Herbal preparations may be used, and regular colon implants of lactobacillus acidophilus are given to assure normalization of bowel flora. Afterwards you may experience improved mental clarity and a greater feeling of well-being.

The Colonic International Association recommends that this treatment is used in conjunction with other therapies.

They say that by improving elimination, response to dietary, homoeopathic, herbal, manipulative and other therapies is markedly improved. Treatments need to be regular over a period of one or two months, and they recommend six-monthly treatment to 'maintain inner cleanliness and good elimination'.

Gillian sufferes from chronic constipation and flatulence. She found that colonic irrigation gave her more of an instant relief from being very constipated than any long-lasting benefit. She says:

'Treatment is not uncomfortable for the most part and lasts about thirty to forty minutes. However, it is expensive – I paid £46 for the first session and £35 subsequently – and practitioners seem to be few and far between, perhaps because inserting tubes in the anal canal and pumping water wouldn't be a job that would appeal to a lot of people!'

Gillian was told that immediately after treatment it is common to empty the bowel thoroughly and sometimes to be constipated again immediately afterwards, which is what happened to her. However, the system then, apparently, readjusts itself. She decided she wouldn't continue with the treatments as, for her, it provided no long-term benefit.

Another patient who suffered from severe constipation – going for as long as two weeks without having a bowel movement – was simply advised by his specialist to take laxatives if he didn't have a bowel movement for more than five days. The laxatives, however, didn't work. He had heard about colonic irrigation and made some enquiries. He takes up the tale:

'I took my courage in my hands and made an appointment! It was one of the wisest things I had done – the relief! He gave me about eight treatments – two a week for two weeks and weekly afterwards, put me on a course of herbs and psyllium husks, lots of water and it has made such a difference.'

Aromatherapy

Aromatherapy uses essential oils, which are extracted from the roots, stalks, flowers, leaves or fruit of a plant, to heal the body. For thousands of years people have used aromatic oils to soothe, relax, create spiritual atmospheres, and protect from infection. The modern form of aromatherapy is about thirty years old.

The odour of essential oils can influence the state of mind. They can also help to reinforce the immune system and have antibacterial, antiseptic and disinfectant properties.

The essential oils are combined with vegetable oils and used in massage, put in the bath or heated in special burners, to create a regenerative and healing effect on the body. Aromatherapy can be especially beneficial in easing stress and anxiety.

As with most practitioners of complementary medicine, a qualified aromatherapist will start by taking a detailed history of your health and lifestyle. Useful oils for treating IBS might include lavender, clary sage, neroli, jasmine, marigold, vetivert (all good for anxiety); eucalyptus, juniper, black pepper, lavender, rosemary (may help to ease pain); rosemary, juniper, black pepper, fennel (may help constipation); lavender, neroli (massage with these can ease diarrhoea and stomach cramps) and peppermint (good for digestive problems).

Essential oils contain potent substances and should only be blended by a qualified aromatherapist. Certain oils should not be used in pregnancy (these include hyssop, marjoram and myrrh), or for babies and very young children, Oils for use on elderly people should be diluted to half strength.

Florence felt uncertain on her first visit to an aromatherapist but found it to be a very enjoyable experience:

'I had been suffering from pain for some time. Someone I met just by chance told me she had been going to an aromatherapist for chronic headaches, and she said she was much improved afterwards. She also said the aromatherapist was qualified and belonged to the International Federation of Aromatherapists and also the British School of Reflexology. Amazingly, she said she paid £30 for three hours. I made an appointment with her – she said to leave three hours for the first session. She spent half an hour taking my medical history, asking about illnesses, feelings, family members, etc. Then she explained that she was going to make up the oils for the massage based on the information I had given her. She spent a few minutes doing this, and then asked me to smell the oils to see if they were acceptable to me – I didn't like the smell of the first oil, and so she adjusted it with other oils, to one which I did like. I then undressed down to my underwear, she covered me with towels and I lay on the special couch. The room was fairly dark, and it was all very discreet. She massaged my back and neck, then covered these parts with a towel, and then started on another part of my body. So for those people who are a bit nervous of a massage, they have nothing to worry about. Your body is covered up, and only exposed bit by bit! Although I was anxious at first, I soon relaxed, and when she had finished I realized another two and a half hours had elapsed! I was so relaxed it was hard to get up and drive home. I went again the next week; it was only £25 this time, but it still lasted two and a half hours. This time I enjoyed it more because I wasn't anxious as I knew what was going to happen and she was no longer a stranger to me. I think it did help with the pain. I have only been three times so far but each time I have felt good afterwards and I feel positive it has benefits for me. I wondered how I could spare three hours for this, but on the other hand, it makes me relax for this time, whereas otherwise I would probably be rushing around. I don't know that it would help people whose IBS had been caused by medical problems, but I'm sure it helps people who are stressed out. I also don't know what part the oils play – I think it might be the actual massage which helps most. I know £25 is a lot of money, and I certainly couldn't afford to go every week, but I am going to try to go every month – I am lucky to have a good job to be able to afford this.'

Bach Flower Remedies

Edward Bach, a renowned Harley street physician and bacteriologist, developed his method of Flower Healing in the 1930s.

The remedies are presecribed not for the physical complaint, but for the patient's state of mind and mood. The principle behind the Bach Flower Remedies is that negative and inharmonious states of mind will not only hinder healing and recovery, but are the primary cause of sickness and disease. For instance, someone who is extremely fearful or anxious will have their vitality depleted. The body loses its natural resistance to disease and the person becomes vulnerable to infection and illness. Edward Bach said: 'There is no true healing unless there is a change in outlook, peace of mind and inner happiness.'

All the remedies are derived from the flowers of wild plants, bushes or trees. None of them is harmful or habit-forming or has any side effects. A few drops of the remedy are taken in a little water.

According to your moods and emotions, you might be prescribed rock rose for terror or extreme fear; aspen for vague fears of an unknown origin; gorse for feelings of hopelessness and despair; pine for feelings of guilt; or vervain for tension and over-enthusiasm. The composite remedy, Rescue Remedy, was formulated for use in emergencies. It is composed of five remedies for shock, terror and panic, mental stress, desperation and for the faraway feeling which often precedes loss of consciousness.

Bach Flower Remedies are often used in conjunction with other therapies.

An Overview

How Does Complementary Medicine Differ from Traditional Western Medicine?

There are significant differences in the way holistic and allopathic medicine look at health and disease. Holistic medicine aims to maintain health; illness is seen as a deviation from health. Allopathic medicine, on the other hand, is preoccupied with disease, and health is taken to be a deviance from disease. In orthodox medicine, diagnosis is of primary importance. Within complementary medicine, diagnosis is of lesser importance; instead, signs and symptoms are noted (including pulse-taking, observing body language, dietary habits, etc.) so that a whole picture can be built up.

In western medical research there is often talk of the 'placebo effect'. A placebo is a supposedly inactive substance or procedure which is often looked upon as a nuisance factor which researchers have to account for when assessing their results. Sometimes, when people's health is improved by complementary medicine, it is dismissed as 'just the result of a placebo effect', and therefore somehow unreal or inferior. However, for many complementary therapists the aim is, as A. V. Conway puts it,

> to bring patients into a position where they have more choice in the beliefs that they have about themselves, and as a result of exercising that choice, and changing their beliefs about themselves, they get better. It is unclear why this subtle, natural and cooperative process should be considered somehow inferior to treatment where a patient has something 'done' (medication, surgery etc.) to him, to 'make' him better. The placebo effect can be extremely powerful . . . Placebos do not just help people feel better, they can dramatically affect physiology ('Assessment of Complementary Medicine: Revolution or Evolution', *Journal of Complementary Medicine*)

Within complementary medicine there is often more of a desire to see the patient as the 'expert' when it comes to their own health. The practitioners are interested in the patient's explanation of their problem and, to some extent, their reasoning behind it, as well as their ideas and reasoning about what should be done. Often the practitioner will have to take up and discuss 'hints' from the patient, especially if they are not used to discussing their health in this cooperative way. Learning how the patient sees their own problem may also be helpful to the practitioner when deciding on treatment. Having said this, the practitioner will not usually see the patient and him or herself as having the same expertise. After all, it is the practitioner who has been consulted for help and advice.

Probably the major difference between the two ways of thinking is that while orthodox medicine attempts to destroy or suppress what is believed to be causing the illness, through drugs, surgery or radiation, complementary medicine seeks to defeat disease by strengthening the whole person's defences.

Here's how C. W. Aakster, in a Dutch study on complementary medicine contrasted the two approaches:

If a disease is something with a non-understandable Latin name, which can only be measured by experts and which can only be cured by doctors, who know the solutions, the doctor is by definition someone who should have had at least seven years of university training, a man (rather than a woman) with great authority (expertness), who takes the lead in the patient's problem solving. If, however, diagnosis is of the functional type, and the therapeutic measures are of a rather simple nature and require the full and active cooperation of the patient (a profound change of dietary habits, regular exercise, etc.) then medicine becomes more manageable. It reverts to the patient and may lead to deprofessionalization, by merely emphasizing basic rules for healthy living, the responsibility of the patient . . .

seeing the person as an integrated whole, as the patient sees himself. ('Concepts in Alternative Medicine', *Journal of Complementary Medicine*)

In addition, most complementary practitioners and their patients choose such disciplines because they want to avoid the harm done by drugs which aren't compatible with the body and cause side effects; painful diagnostic tests; and mutilating operations.

Others, however, may choose alternative medicine because they see it as having almost mystical qualities and may be attracted to it because of this. If they are helped, all well and good; but these people may be particularly vulnerable to ineffective or even charlatan practitioners.

A criticism sometimes made is that some people seek out complementary treatments as a last-ditch attempt, a clutching at straws, after orthodox medicine has failed them. Again, the sceptics say, these people may be easily taken advantage of. The answer to these criticisms, of course, is better regulation of complementary practitioners and the availability of their treatment on the NHS, or at low rates, so that patients are protected.

The Wind of Change?

Much of twentieth-century medical science in the west has based its thinking on the idea that a disease is a distinct entity (a 'thing'), separate from the person who has the disease. Traditional research methods have also emerged from this perspective, which is one of the reasons why it is difficult to evaluate complementary medicine using such methods. There is some indication however, that this may be changing and that a more holistic way of conducting research may be developing. Dr David St George, senior lecturer in clinical epidemiology at the Royal Free Hospital School of Medicine in London, has this to say: 'Research is being undertaken to explore the new holistic paradigm. If this shift is really taking place – and I personally believe it is – we are right in the middle of it, and no one has a full picture of how it will emerge.' Explaining what this would mean, he goes on to say:

> The body would no longer be seen as an impersonal bi-molecular machine, but as a multi-layered hierarchical system with consciousness at its core. Disease would be seen to arise from different levels within the hierarchy and treatment would focus on self-correction, using the therapist as an external catalyst, stimulus or mirror, rather than focusing exclusively on external bio-engineering.

Dr St George also believes that complementary medical research should equally focus on basic scientific research into the theories and mechanisms which underpin the various methods.

It is clear that there is a growing interest in complementary therapies among some sections of the allopathic medical profession. In this country there are already more than 300 GPs who practise acupuncture and 250 who use homoeopathy; and many are osteopaths. Nurses, in particular, are taking courses in massage, nutrition (it is ironic that this should be needed in addition to the basic training), aromatherapy, reflexology and counselling. The British Medical Association has called for a 'familiarization course' on complementary medicine to be included within the medical undergraduate curriculum.

During the research I did for this chapter, it was clear that many sufferers were satisfied with the way they were dealt with by complementary therapists, sometimes in favourable comparison with the approach of doctors and specialists. They often cited the thorough case histories that were taken, the caring and sympathetic attitudes – and, of particular importance to IBS sufferers, the feeling that they were being taken seriously, sometimes for the first time.

It was also clear, however, that complementary medicine, as a whole, cannot guarantee to help IBS sufferers. There are some positive cases, where the sufferer's IBS has been virtually eliminated; but more often relief is only temporary, and symptoms return after treatment stops, or the relief experienced is minor, vague or elusive. Some sufferers in this position may find it hard to break away from receiving the treatment, hoping that they will get better but at the same time wondering how much they are being helped. This dilemma can be particularly acute in view of the large amounts of money that are sometimes being spent.

Philippa, who suffers from abdominal pain with bloating and vomiting, says:

'In desperation I tried some alternative remedies, to no avail. I went to a homoeopath, who thought it was a gynaecological problem, and an osteopath, who said it might be the appendix. Confused? So am I!'

And Moira, who is 50 and has had IBS for over twenty years, was not helped by the treatments she tried:

'I have not found orthodox or alternative therapies very helpful. I have read widely on the subject and tried everything suggested without much success. I was managing a health food shop when my problem began and had been involved with alternative therapies for some time. I felt very guilty when natural methods I would advocate for others had no effect on me!'

On a more positive note, complementary medicine has a well-deserved reputation for increasing a person's sense of well-being and overall health. Many therapies are pleasant and extremely relaxing. IBS sufferers often say, even if their symptoms remain, that they feel better able to cope with their condition.

It is clear that no one therapy stands out as being particularly beneficial to IBS sufferers. Potentially, all may have something to offer; but you need to be able to make an informed choice. A great deal depends on the individual practitioner, and, of course, on you as the patient. As Dr Christine Page, who is both a medical doctor and a homoeopath, says:

'I don't think that homoeopathy is unique. Many therapies look at the whole person and most work towards restoring balance and not just suppressing symptoms, as with orthodox treatment. The patient eventually makes the decision and will be attracted to one form of therapy more than another. Sometimes personal recommendation will sway them in one direction. There is no therapy better than another and it depends very much on the therapist and the patient rather than the therapy. Orthodox medicine also has its place and can be used if necessary in harmony with complementary care.'

And the last word goes to Gillian, who has tried various different forms of complementary medicine:

'It is apparent from my own and [others] experiences that different treatments work differently for different people and that there is no one effective treatment to suit everyone. I imagine that one's personal belief system about a particular treatment may well have a positive part to play in the outcome as well. At the very least, it must surely help to suspend judgement and keep an open mind – however merely believing in a particular form of treatment (a kind of placebo effect) doesn't seem to be enough in itself to guarantee an effective outcome! But, I think, the opposite – not believing in a treatment at all – would probably be sufficient to ensure it has little chance or potential to help!'

7

Help Yourself to Health: The Role of Self-help Groups in Treating IBS

Christine P. Dancey ★

'I believe the IBS Network is pioneering nothing short of a revolution in health care and that the medical profession should lend their support to this initiative.' (Professor Nick Read, Northern General Hospital, Sheffield)

'Self-help' refers to help which is initiated by the patients, or, in this case, by IBS sufferers themselves. In other words, you may get together with other sufferers from IBS and decide how best to help yourselves. You may want to do this by setting up small discussion groups, to inform and support each other. Together, you may decide to set up telephone helplines or befriender groups, or to communicate with each other by newsletter or letter-writing. These are all forms of self-help: the common theme is that the activities are initiated and organized by the people themselves rather than by professionals such as doctors or health projects.

What Are Self-Help Groups?

Groups which are formed for the purpose of sharing personal experiences of a particular problem, and for giving mutual support and information, are called self-help groups, or

★ The author would like to thank the medical practitioners and coordinators of the IBS self-help groups who contributed to this chapter by giving their views on self-help.

support groups. One 1989 study revealed that in 1987 there were 6.25 million members of self-help groups, over age seventeen, in the USA, a figure predicted to rise to 10 million by 1999. Unfortunately, there has been no comparable research into overall numbers of self-help groups in Britain. However, a spokeswoman at the Self Help Centre in London (now, sadly, closed down) said that self-help groups are a growing phenomenon: for instance, in Nottingham in 1982 there were 82 groups, and in 1994 there were 165. Groups now exist for most chronic diseases: there are hundreds of distinct groups, for conditions such as Alzheimer's, diabetes, cancer, tranquillizer addiction, alcoholism, impotence, hysterectomies and bereavement, to name but a few – and, since 1991, for IBS.

Self-help groups have been defined as 'usually formed by peers who have come together for mutual assistance in satisfying a common need, overcoming a common handicap or life-disrupting problem, and bringing about social and/or personal change'. This definition is particularly suitable to the groups which have been formed by IBS sufferers. They have generally come together in order to help each other deal with the physical symptoms and the psychological and social effects of Irritable Bowel Syndrome, which, while not life-threatening, can be very disruptive of normal life. As a sufferer of IBS, particularly if you are a long-time sufferer, you may realize that your symptoms could remain with you for some time, and you may need support in coping with them. Rather than allowing your symptoms to overwhelm you, you need to be able somehow to keep them in the background. This is the personal change which you, as an IBS sufferer, need, which can help you while you wait for social and medical change to come about – social change in the form of better knowledge of the problem and acceptance for IBS sufferers, and medical change in the form of better treatment and increased facilities for people with bowel problems.

Since groups are usually formed by the sufferers themselves, they are based on trust and reciprocity; IBS groups generally have no 'leader', being rather a group of people who act together as equals; if professionals are involved, they usually take on a minor role. Basically, such groups are run by the sufferers, for the sufferers. This is generally the case with groups of sufferers of any chronic disease or disorder.

Self-help groups may have been seen in the past as something peripheral, which *might* help, and could at least do no harm. However, such groups have gained acceptance over the years as a valid form of health care. Self-help groups are often set up in order to meet a need which is not being met by the NHS:

'So many people suffer from IBS, far more than the Health Service can cope with. The situation is made worse by the fact that medical treatments for IBS seem not to be very effective for a large number of patients.' (Professor Nick Read, Northern General Hospital, Sheffield)

Although self-help groups are run by the sufferers them-selves, this does not mean that they cannot make use of medical expertise. Professionals often wish to work *with* self-help groups, rather than against them. In fact, professionals can assist self-help groups by referring people to them. Dr Chris Mallinson, consultant physician at the Lewisham Hospital NHS Trust in south London, says:

'I do find it helpful to have the IBS Network at hand. It has to be said that quite a lot of patients don't want to know about it to begin with but increasingly we are able to put patients in touch.'

Other medical practitioners find that self-help groups can keep them in touch with what their patients think:

'I have found the newsletter of the IBS Network to be useful in giving me some feedback on what patients think. One worry about talking to patients as a physician is that they are often guarded in expressing thoughts and opinions, and therefore, it is useful to have some inside information on what patients tell each other. Reassuringly, the concerns that are expressed are very similar to those that I hear.' (Professor David Wingate, The London Hospital Medical College)

These sentiments are echoed by Professor Michael Farthing of St Bartholomew's Hospital, London:

'Publications like those of the IBS Network are useful for healthworkers as they often present the "patient's perspective" in a succinct and direct way.'

IBS groups often initiate contact with professionals, in order to use their expertise. Professionals can help with accommodation for groups; they can speak to the group regularly and keep them up-to-date with information, give them advice and perhaps write occasional articles for newsletters. However, group members generally prefer that professionals stay in the background, being non-directive and non-authoritarian.

What Are Self-Help Groups Like?

Self-help groups in general differ in numbers, outlook and the way they run the meetings. IBS groups also differ, as each group is autonomous; that is, there is no one body which 'controls' local groups. Local IBS self-help groups are generally small, with between five and eight members at any one meeting, although often there are twenty or thirty people 'on the books'; some even have as many as forty-five people listed, although this is rare at present. Although some groups do not hold meetings (they talk to each other on the phone instead, or write letters), most meet once a month, or once every two months, usually at the home of one of the members. Some groups meet in a room made available to them by their local GP or hospital. Most groups started up by advertising for members in their local newspaper.

'We first met together in April 1992 and now meet about every two to three months at my home. We make it as positive, friendly, relaxed and informal as possible. The members of the group vary as symptoms and other commitments permit, but we usually average about six each time.' (South-West Hertfordshire group coordinator)

'The Exmouth and East Devon IBS Support Group was started in March 1992 at my home with just a few interested sufferers. We now have over forty-five members and we meet monthly at Exmouth Hospital, where we have either a speaker or a general discussion. Members represent a good cross-section of the community and are of all ages, both male and female, from all over Devon.' (Exmouth and East Devon group coordinator)

How Can an IBS Group Help You?

'The major reason for a [support] group is to give hope, encouragement and support, especially as illness can seem very lonely – as if you are the only person in the world who suffers this way.' (Ian Forgacs, consultant at King's College Hospital, Dulwich)

People with IBS often ask their doctors, or the IBS Network, how such groups can help them. Sometimes people phrase their questions in such a way that they seem prejudiced against such groups from the start; some, for example, ask: 'How can a bunch of people moaning about their symptoms help get themselves better?' Others say: 'How can a group help me when the doctors themselves don't know how to help?' You may be reading this book now, wondering how meeting with a group of like-minded people could actually help you physically. Comments such as those quoted above show that the questioner feels that the only purpose of treatment is to relieve her/his symptoms directly, and also that the questioner has not considered that there might be a relationship between emotional and social support, and symptoms.

Large numbers of people are finding that by organizing themselves into groups they can help themselves in all sorts of ways. Self-help groups cannot alleviate symptoms in a direct manner, so anybody who comes to a group thinking that their symptoms will be relieved just by attending the group will be sadly disappointed. However, self-help groups *can* help indirectly. As you no doubt realize, symptoms are made worse by stress, anxiety and lack of support from partners, friends, family and so on. Participants in studies researching IBS often say that stress makes their IBS worse. Indeed, anxiety and stress make *any* illness worse, not just IBS. So if you can manage to lessen your anxiety, and not feel so stressed about having IBS (and all sufferers understand how difficult this is), while your symptoms may not go away completely, they may be somewhat alleviated. Through reading this chapter, you will see that being part of a self-help group for IBS can help you with the stress and anxiety which you may find accompanies the condition.

This is how Professor Nick Read sees self-help groups as being of benefit to IBS sufferers:

'There is a need to break the mould and explore new methods of managing IBS. It is here that the IBS Network and IBS self-help groups are such an important initiative. The treatment of IBS requires a holistic approach that involves psychology, nutrition, an examination of lifestyle, exercise, as well as medical factors. To go into all of this requires much more time than the average doctor has at his/her disposal. I believe that the most effective means by which the medical profession can tackle the epidemic of IBS is to encourage the establishment of a network of self-help groups throughout the country and to work closely with these groups to educate and facilitate the support of their members. It is not that the treatment of IBS is difficult, it's more that it requires insight into the way in which life events, stress, food and other factors all interact to produce disturbances in bowel function. These principles can be taught to sufferers of IBS who through the self-help groups can produce a network of support and confidence.'

What Benefits Will You Gain by Joining a Group?

Researchers have tried to find out how members felt their lives had improved as a result of joining self-help groups. Although this research was not conducted on IBS groups, they would be expected to produce similar benefits. One researcher studied the benefits of self-help groups as depicted by 232 members from 65 different groups. Briefly, he found that:

- 80 per cent experienced an improvement in health;
- three-quarters reported positive changes in other aspects of their lives;
- members participated in social life more actively – half became more enterprising and more outgoing;
- a quarter reported positive changes in their relationships with partners;
- over half said they had greater knowledge of their illness;
- over half made use of that knowledge by being able to deal with medical professionals more effectively;
- three-quarters were able to reduce drug treatments as they learned of other ways of treating themselves.

This same researcher also listed benefits identified by other researchers. One found that 'helping others, help from others, coping strategies, sense of community, coping with public attitudes, factual information, spirit of hope, self-confidence and meeting others with similar problems' all gave benefit to members. In another study, the most frequently mentioned responses were that the group had provided social involvement and fellowship (43 per cent) and a supportive, accepting environment (83 per cent). Another found that 76 per cent said that sharing thoughts and feelings was important, 68 per cent said they felt supported, approved of and valued, and 63 per cent mentioned knowing that their problems, feelings and fears were not unique.

The following sections describe some of the particular benefits gained by people who have joined IBS self-help groups.

'I Know Just How You Feel'

The most immediate benefit is that as a new member, you are able to talk about your symptoms without embarrassment, knowing that the other members will understand what you are going through. Those members who have been in self-help groups for some time are often amazed at the relief expressed by new members when they are able to talk about their symptoms, because they themselves have forgotten what it was like in the beginning, when they had no one to confide in. Most sufferers of IBS do not talk about their condition to their friends or family; if they do confide in someone, it is likely to be just one member of the family, and they try not to talk about it too much. Sufferers often are too embarrassed to talk about their problems. However, as one of the purposes of a self-help group is for members to be able to talk about themselves and their problems, you should feel justified in talking about yourself to others in the group. Thus the immediate benefit for you is to be able to talk – about your symptoms, your problems, and sometimes your anger at people who have not understood your predicament, often doctors and family. Often you may want to talk in depth about your feelings with regard to the medical profession. Talking in a non-judgemental atmosphere and having your views validated can provide an immediate relief.

'I Thought I Was the Only One!'

Interacting in a self-help group relieves the isolation felt by people who previously knew no one with IBS – or rather, *thought* they knew no one: since IBS sufferers try to keep their condition secret, it is often the case that people do know others with the condition but do not realize it! Once people begin talking about their condition, they find that others will say: 'I suffered from that some years ago,' or; 'My sister has IBS really badly.' As IBS has had more publicity in the last few years, so there are many more people who know what it is. Once you have been in a group for some time, you will find you gain confidence, and are able to tell others of your problems. Trying to keep a condition like IBS secret is a source of stress in itself, and being open and honest about yourself relieves some of this stress. Often sufferers feel very alone, and 'abnormal', and this sense of abnormality often leads in turn to a sense of isolation from others. Groups generally act to give members a sense of normality, which they often find they have lost as their symptoms have increased.

'We all talk freely about IBS and its many and varied symptoms without any embarrassment and are able to pass on tips to each other on ways of being able to talk about IBS openly and to be amongst others who know what it is like to suffer from this distressing condition.' (Member of Farnham, Surrey self-help group)

Access to More Information about IBS

People generally join self-help groups because the medical profession has not met their needs in full, and groups can provide information and advice which has not been given by such professionals. Since medical practitioners have a limited amount of time to spend with each patient with IBS, they cannot give each individual all the information s/he needs. When asked what the medical profession could have done to help them the most, IBS sufferers did not cite more or better drugs – they said that what they wanted most was information on IBS. Self-help groups are often able to give this information.

'What I've Found Helps is . . .'

Members are often able to pass on tips on how to cope with particular problems or questions which are troublesome. For example, you may be worrying about whether your symptoms are due to something more serious than IBS – cancer, for instance. Other sufferers will be able to reassure you on this point, with the knowledge they have gained over the past months or years. You may not have had hospital tests to exclude the more serious diseases yet, and you may be worried about going for tests; sometimes sufferers are terrified. Other members can often tell you all about these tests – they have been through them, and survived them. At other times members will be able to give you support and advice in dealing with 'difficult' GPs. Often members feel intimidated by GPs and consultants and unable to put the questions they want to ask. Other members can help you through these problems.

Long-time members are able to share their experiences with you, showing you that they have managed to cope with their IBS, that they still find enjoyment in life, and that their IBS can be put in the background. This is very important, as members tend to join groups when they are feeling at their worst – indeed, this is often why they have joined – because joining a self-help group is sometimes seen as a last resort. This should not be the case; a self-help group really should be the *first* resort, because joining one gives you so many advantages, as members will tell you. Nevertheless, people do often come to groups at their lowest, worn down, depressed and anxious. Talking to long-time members, most of whom have improved over time, can be uplifting. Longtime members can often talk about the things which have helped them through their IBS, both psychological and medical. Often, when discussing which treatments helped them, long-time members are able to point newcomers in a promising direction. You may not have tried, or even thought of, a certain treatment before – members can give you the experience of their advice. Just being able to consider a range of treatments which *may* be beneficial, and which you could try, will give you hope.

'I've Just Read this Great Book'

One of the more popular discussions in IBS groups is about books and articles on IBS that are available. Before 1989 there were hardly any books on IBS that were accessible to the layperson. The first general book on IBS for the layperson was written by Rosemary Nicol in 1989 and is still extremely popular. Two more, published in 1990, were by Geoff Watts and Shirley Trickett; *Overcoming IBS*, written by the editors of this book, was published in 1993. During this time a few specialist books on aspects of IBS have also appeared, for instance on IBS and herbalism (*Herbal Remedies: Irritable Bowel*, 1992) by D Potterton and *Beat IBS through Diet* by the Stewarts, who have written chapter 3 in this book.

Between them, members of self-help groups generally have a good knowledge of these publications and can discuss them with new members, who are then in a better position to choose the book(s) which will suit them. Sometimes self-help groups are able to buy books which they can then lend to members.

'I Thought it was My fault'

Another benefit of self-help groups is that members begin to believe that IBS is a disorder worth taking seriously. So many sufferers have felt that they are to blame for their IBS, and that others blamed them too. Often they feel that IBS is not given as much consideration as other disorders. Many medics try to reassure IBS sufferers that IBS is a definite, positive, valid diagnosis; however, the people whom we have met through the IBS Network do not seem to have this view. Often they feel that their IBS is due to some personality deficit, some inability to cope properly. Members of self-help groups come to believe that IBS is a valid disorder, which should be dealt with properly, rather than a trivial complaint which they should be able to deal with. This helps them cope:

> 'Personally, I find that having a group gives IBS the recognition that it is not something trivial that some people have to deal with.' (Member of Isle of Wight self-help group)

'Now You're Here, Doctor, We'd Like to Ask . . .'

Most self-help groups invite professionals to speak at some of their meetings. Despite not being funded, they have been able to persuade professors of gastroenterology, dietitians specializing in IBS and complementary health practitioners to speak to them.

> 'To date we have had speakers on hypnotherapy, reflexology, aromatherapy, homoeopathy, acupuncture, physiotherapy – also a counsellor and a dietitian, but most of our members find the general discussion meetings of most benefit and our discussions are both varied and informative – it does help to know that one does not suffer alone when GPs seem unable to help.' (Member of East Devon self-help group)

> 'At our meetings we exchange ideas and experiences. Our invited guests have included an osteopath who followed naturopathic practice as advocate of homoeopathy, a much improved sufferer who gave us hope and shared tips and coping strategies with us, and a minister and his wife (a leukaemia sufferer) who helped us to explore how faith can help with chronic health problems. (Member of South-West Hertfordshire self-help group)

Since most IBS self-help groups are quite small, such meetings with professionals are fairly intimate and nonthreatening. Members feel more able to ask questions about their IBS in this sort of setting than in a more formal setting such as a hospital, where they would often feel intimidated.

Also, sufferers have more confidence in a situation such as this because of the support of the others in the group. Gastroenterologists who have taken the opportunity to speak to these small groups have also found that they can talk in a friendly, relaxed way, more so than they would find appropriate in their consulting rooms.

> 'I think the visit to the local group emphasized what a tremendously broad network a group of this sort provides. It would have been almost impossible to categorize the patients that I met, given their variety of age and experience of IBS. Nevertheless a thread runs through the group, as indeed it does through the comments in the articles in *Gut Reaction* [the IBS newsletter], which I read with interest – one of the threads being the complete lack of unanimity about any sort of treatment.' (Dr Chris Mallinson, Lewisham Hospital NHS Trust, south London)

'It Helps to Know Someone's There'

All the above points relate to social and emotional support. Many sufferers do not feel they have support from the medical profession, friends or families. Many keep their problems secret from others, especially their employers. Members of a group can help each other through mutual support – giving a shoulder to lean on, being at the end of a phone in times of crisis. Even when a member is unable to attend a local self-help group, just knowing others are there, suffering from the same type of problems, gives them a sense of support.

> 'Perhaps our most important achievement has been the instigation of a local telephone contact list which enables us to help a much wider circle of sufferers who are either unable or unwilling to attend meetings.
> 'We have all found it very helpful to have the opportunity to share our concerns with others who really understand and are not shocked, embarrassed or judgemental about our condition. We don't have to keep "pretending".

'Instead of feeling isolated and ashamed we feel reassured that there is always a friendly voice at the end of a telephone if needed and a ready supply of advice about treatments tried as well as ongoing updates of recent research from those currently undergoing specialist treatment.' (Member of South-West Hertfordshire self-help group)

Making Friends

Some people in groups become close friends and see each other outside of group meetings, and some studies have shown that members who develop these out-of-group activities have a greater sense of well-being than people who do not do this. Of course, it could be that people who feel a greater sense of well-being are more likely to make friends and see each other outside of the group anyway.

'I have made many new friends. I know that the self-help group I created has helped me so much. I have people I can talk to when I have a bad attack of IBS.' (Coordinator, High Wycombe self-help group)

Benefits for the Long-Time Member

The preceding sections have concentrated on the benefits of group membership from the point of view of the new member. But how do groups benefit the long-time member? After all, long-time members will have spoken about their symptoms and IBS-related problems, and generally feel no need to go over the same ground repeatedly. However, their need for emotional and social support, while it may have lessened during the time they have been in the group, will still be there. Also, such members feel a sense of satisfaction in knowing they are of help to new, less secure members.

In theory it is probably easier to see the benefits of relying on others for advice and support than to see how helping others can benefit you directly. Yet in 1988 a researcher who studied three different kinds of self-help groups (not

IBS) found that people who *both* gave *and* received support were less depressed, and found greater benefits and group satisfaction, than people who *only* gave support, or *only* received it!

'I take telephone calls from sufferers when they are feeling down. Just having someone to talk to helps a lot. I now have over thirty sufferers on my database who I write to every three months. I have great support from the Priory Centre, High Wycombe.' (Coordinator, High Wycombe self-help group)

Beginning to Look Outward

Long-time members, having made friends, often feel a sense of belonging, and often feel the need to keep the group going most strongly. The needs and interests of such members are different from those of new entrants: perhaps not needing any more to talk about themselves, or requiring crisis intervention, they often begin to look outward from the group, and to focus on bettering the lot of IBS sufferers in general. In other words, once you feel more confident of yourself and are able to feel secure in your own coping mechanisms for IBS, then you are able to move forward to helping in a more general sense. For instance, some members want to help raise the profile of the condition by talking to other groups about IBS, or by writing to their local MPs about toilet facilities in public places, or by offering to talk to the media about IBS – in other words, raising the political profile of IBS. Over the past three years, two members of IBS Network groups have been on television to talk about their IBS, and four have given telephone interviews for women's magazines. Such activities benefit all IBS sufferers and as such are likely to be a source of satisfaction to members, which in turn increases their own confidence and self-esteem.

Clare, the previous coordinator of the Wandsworth group, decided to speak out about her IBS on a London television programme, *Capital Woman*, for several reasons. Here she explains exactly what these were:

'I was hoping that the four-minute slot on *Capital Woman* might lead to a whole programme devoted to IBS – there was so much more I wanted to say – I needed four hours not four minutes!

I agreed to do the programme because I was tired of reading about how IBS is a stress-related illness. Personally, the only stress I have is the illness itself. I wanted the world to know just how awful IBS is, and I wanted people to actually *see* that I really look quite ordinary – I don't have green skin with purple spots, I'm not neurotic and externally I look well. The more people who know about IBS the better chance we have about finding the answer. Maybe more doctors will become interested and take up the challenge of finding out what it is and how to put it right. I'm not prepared to take this lying down. I'm going to go on talking about it, writing about it, whatever it takes, until the answer is found.'

What Self-Help Groups Can't Do

Self-help groups cannot cure IBS. One of the reasons for some people feeling that groups cannot help them is that they start with unrealistic expectations of the group – they are hoping it will mean their symptoms will disappear.

Some members often feel too ill to travel to a meeting, especially as some groups are thinly scattered. For instance, the coordinator of the North-West London group says:

'I read at the weekend in an article on ME self-help groups – "We are the only self-help group that nobody attends as we are all too sick to get there." I know what the writer means and I sympathize with her, but I think if people make the effort to get to a meeting it may be of reward to them and to us.'

It is true that some people may not gain much from a self-help group. These are usually people who are different in certain respects from the rest of the members: for example, occasionally a sufferer is referred to a group with a diagnosis of IBS but has symptoms very different from the rest of the group. Betty was referred to a London self-help group as an IBS sufferer by a local GP. When talking to her, the group found that she suffered from nausea but had no abdominal pain and no bowel problems – yet her GP had told her that she suffered from IBS. Although the group in question were very sympathetic to Betty, and tried to help her, it was clear that she was very different from the rest of the group and felt out of place. The more similar you are to the rest of the group, the more likely you are to feel part of it, and therefore benefit from it.

Professor Wingate feels that self-help groups are not beneficial to everyone. He says:

'A problem shared . . .' may be true and there is no doubt that some patients benefit. I do not think that this is true of all patients and there are some theoretical or even actual negative aspects . . . affiliation to a patient network could mean, for some people, affiliation to a state of chronic invalidism. This is, of course, true of other conditions; a crutch can either be used as a badge of disability or an accessory to enable its owner to lead a normal life.'

However, Professor Wingate feels that the advantages outweigh the disadvantages:

'On balance, I believe that self-help groups are a good thing because they underline the autonomy of patients. They also lift some of the burdens of looking after this disorder from physicians.'

Funding

Since self-help groups are meeting a definite need in the community, and are supporting care by the NHS, I believe that such groups should be supported by grants from local councils or health authorities. Self-help groups are perceived as having a wide range of benefits by the people who attend them, and no doubt help some people who would otherwise use the NHS to a greater extent. Given adequate finance, self-help groups could perhaps be involved in preventative work rather than dealing primarily with sufferers when they are at their lowest.

At present, however, most groups are largely self-supporting. All such groups need funds in order to exist – for basic needs such as tea, coffee and biscuits, and also for more costly items such as stationery and postage, telephone calls, and paying travelling expenses to speakers. Often group members contribute subscriptions to help with running costs, but still most groups are low on funds:

> 'We have no funds as such but to raise money for postage, refreshments, etc. at the last few meetings each member has brought a small item to raffle and this helps with costs. Our members are very keen to keep the group going, but like all groups we need new members with new ideas.'
> (Member of Essex self-help group)

With adequate finances groups can be proactive – they can recruit more effectively, they can publicize their existence much more widely (through the Family Practitioners Committee, for instance; charges vary, but it can cost £25 for them to send out your literature to the doctors in their area) and they can disseminate information to the general public by leaflets and posters through stalls at charity fairs. Groups can use such funds for speakers who make a charge for their time, and for buying copies of IBS-related books to lend to members. All such activities cost money, and groups could do so much more if they had funding.

If you start a group, or already belong to one, it is worth writing to your local council to ask whether any grants exist to help your group get off the ground. One IBS group did this (Sydenham, in south London) and in 1991 was awarded

£1,000 from Lewisham Council, enabling it to buy books for members to borrow, to have their literature sent out to all GPs in the borough, to buy stamps, stationery, etc. and to pay speakers' expenses – and generally not to worry about finance for some time to come.

Belonging to a National Organization

'I'm a new member and when I started reading all the newsletters I cried, I cried, what a relief I'm not going mad after all.' (Letter to IBS Network, 1994)

Often local organizations are 'held together' by a parent organization, that is, a national body which produces a newsletter and gives advice and support to individuals and local groups. This is the case with, for instance, NACC (National Association for Crohn's Disease and Colitis), the ME Association (for myalgic encephalitis) and the Endometriosis Society, as well as the IBS Network. Groups such as these produce regular newsletters, with contributions from professionals and members. Members may or may not wish to join a local self-help group, and many do not; often, people just do not feel the need to join a local group, but wish to receive information and advice from the parent organization. This is the case with the IBS Network. Despite the absence of personal contact which the self-help group can give you, you will still feel that you 'belong' to an organization which supports and cares for you:

'. . . as all sufferers will heartily agree, IBS is depressing, painful, embarrassing and little researched, or so it would appear. That is why most of us welcome all the help we can give to and receive from others. This Society seems to be well organized and to fulfil a long-felt need. Shared experiences can provide not only ourselves, but also the medical profession with valuable information.' (Letter in *Gut Reaction*, no. 11)

Also, a quarterly newsletter can give you information, advice and the knowledge that there are hundreds of people with exactly the same problems as you have. Just knowing that there are other people who are coping with IBS should make you feel less isolated.

'What a wonderful power for good you have created. *Gut Reaction* is such a help. You have turned the ignorance, pain, trauma and despair of IBS into something we can now come to grips with – because we are sharing it! To read of others mind-blowing problems helps us deal with our own, and we no longer feel freaks. Thank you.' (Letter in *Gut Reaction*, no.12)

Members know there are the opportunities for them to join in self-help groups or befriending schemes (discussed later in this chapter), if they so wish, and this in itself makes them feel more secure.

Starting a Group

You may want to join a group, but find there isn't one in your area. If you are thinking of starting a group, the first thing to do is to think about premises. Do you want to have the group meet at your home? There are definite advantages in this. The home is generally a more comfortable environment for people to meet in than a doctor's surgery, hospital or community flat. Also, you do not need to go out at night to your meeting! However, some people prefer somewhere more neutral to meet. You could ask your GP whether s/he has a spare room that you could use for your meetings, or make contact with the consultant in the gastroenterology department of your local hospital, which may be able to offer you a room in which to meet. Otherwise, try to find an advice centre or voluntary organization in your area, and ask their advice. The advantages to having somewhere like this to meet are, of course, that your group will be able to take it in turns to open up, make the coffee, etc., and you may be able to share the responsibility for the group. Also, groups which meet in hospitals seem to be more successful in terms of numbers – maybe this is because people perceive groups like this as having more 'validity' because they are seen to be backed up by the medical profession!

Once you have somewhere to meet, then you need to find a few people to come to your first meeting. Set a date and time for the first meeting. Ring or write to your local newspaper telling them what you are doing. Put up posters in your GP's surgery, health stores, and libraries. (The IBS Network can help you with posters.) Make sure everyone is clear about the place, date and time. Decide how long you are going to meet for – most groups meet for one and a half to two hours. Organize refreshments, and have a rough idea about what you want to do.

The first meeting is the easiest; people want to introduce themselves, and talk through their symptoms and problems. You will want to discuss what everyone wants out of the group, possible speakers, and other issues relating to the actual running of the group. Be sure to set a definite date and time for the next meeting.

If you are thinking of joining a new group or setting up one yourself, it is important not to imagine that everyone setting up groups has experience in these matters, is efficient and knows what they are doing! Most people who set up groups have had absolutely no experience of setting up or running a group. They took the plunge, and managed. So can you!

Successful Groups

In research on self-help groups, three things were identified by one researcher, K. I. Maton, as especially important in successful groups. These are:
- the role each member plays;
- rules and regulations
- core members.

The Role Each Member Plays

If each member has a clearly defined role – for instance, one person makes the tea, another organizes the speakers, another greets new members and so on, each member will feel a greater commitment to the group. Maton found, too, that in groups which were run like this, members had a greater sense of well-being. Also, the coordinator of an IBS group is less likely to leave if they feel supported in what they are doing.

Rules and Regulations

According to Maton, a certain amount of organization at meetings is necessary if members are actually to benefit from them. For some groups, this may mean following a set agenda rather than having members just chat about anything which comes to mind.

Rules and regulations can be minimal, but they should exist. For instance, one self-help group for sufferers of multiple sclerosis has eleven guidelines which they believe help the group to survive. These are:

- This self-help group belongs to you, and its success rests largely with you.
- Enter into the discussions enthusiastically.
- Give freely of your experiences.
- Confine your discussion to the problem being dealt with.
- Say what you think.
- Only one person should talk at a time.
- Avoid private conversation while someone else is speaking.
- Be patient with other members.
- Appreciate the other person's point of view.
- Do not break confidentiality. If you do, you will be asked to leave the group.
- A member must attend at least one regular self-help group meeting between socials to qualify to attend the socials.

Some people may feel they prefer the group to just meet and chat, but with no clear sense of direction many groups lose members, fail to recruit, and eventually close down.

Core Members

Although members of a self-help group have equal responsibility, it does seem that only a few individuals in each group 'lead' (or perhaps do the work!). Such people are important in the group, because they often have an important influence on group organization; so it is important that such 'core' members are capable.

Coordinators often complain that it is easy to set up a group, but harder to keep it going. Groups must continually recruit new members if they are to survive as other members eventually leave. Also, if group coordinators take too much responsibility for the group, others can become dependent on them: the coordinator may then feel s/he is doing too much, may become ill or just plain fed up, and may no longer want to be involved. Also, others in the group feel a lessening of responsibility for the group, as they have no hand in running it.

To ensure that the group remains of interest to everyone, the members need to discuss every so often what they want out of the group. Most individuals in groups want expert speakers. This involves work – finding out which professionals have an interest in IBS, writing to them, maintaining contact with them and asking them to speak at the group is a task in itself. Once the speaker has agreed to come at a set time, people in the group need to organize publicity – perhaps posters in local surgeries and libraries – arrange for refreshments and make sure everything is running smoothly on the night. Nothing is more embarrassing than turning up with an invited speaker and finding only two people have arrived, due to a series of mishaps.

Everyone needs to be encouraged to do something, so that there is a feeling of togetherness.

Befriending Schemes and Penpals

Sometimes it has not been possible to set up a group in a particular area of the country, despite a willing coordinator and good publicity. This is no fault of the people who try to set up groups. Setting up a group, and keeping it running, on limited resources can be quite difficult. Some people have found they have had an enormous response to local advertising – quite often coordinators find they have twenty or thirty replies to a small piece in the local newspaper, and other members wanting to join through seeing publicity in doctors' surgeries, libraries and so on. Other coordinators, despite doing everything possible, are not so lucky:

> 'I tried, I really did. I had publicity in the free local paper covering thousands of homes, I put adverts in shops in my village and the surrounding villages, and of the dozen names supplied by the IBS Network only one was willing or able to come. Many reasons were given, but basically the north-east is just too vast an area to host a self-help group. You need lots of more localized groups. Trying to find a venue for a meeting when members live sixty miles apart is virtually impossible, but that is the state at the moment. If anyone wants to ring me, or write to me, that is fine. In actual fact I have started writing to a lady who sounded very desperate in her first letter to me, and much appreciated the letter I wrote back to her. It seemed to end her sense of isolation in trying to cope with a condition that is so embarrassing to talk about. I was also contacted by another lady who asked if I could give her any advice, or indeed minded if she started a group of her own. In actual fact she helped me more than I helped her. I hope to meet this lady soon to see if we can organize a Newcastle based group. Anyway, if we manage to do that I will be delighted.'

This coordinator was obviously very disappointed that her efforts were seemingly unrewarded. However, although she has not managed to start a group yet, with continued publicity she may eventually be able to do so.

Sometimes, as in the case of the coordinator quoted above, although it is not possible to start or continue a self-help group, contacts are made by telephone or letter which offer support to those involved. In the example above, the coordinator has found a source of support in the couple of other people she has contacted, and these people will also benefit from her experience. Other coordinators have also found themselves (accidentally!) acting as befrienders while attempting to set up a group.

Sometimes befriending schemes are the support network of choice for many people. There are several reasons why some sufferers prefer befriending schemes to group meetings, including:

- they are not able or willing to travel large distances, often at night, in order to attend a group;
- they prefer one-to-one contact;
- they prefer to be more anonymous.

The befriending schemes run by the IBS Network are essentially different from penpal schemes in that befrienders offer the benefit of their experience and advice to someone who tends to be newly diagnosed as having IBS, and who feels they need contact with someone who is coping well with IBS, in order to see them through the bad times. The befriending schemes that are run for IBS sufferers tend to work by post or phone, since there are not enough befrienders or befriendees to match people up according to area. Neither are befrienders or befriendees matched on other qualities, again unlike penpal schemes. Such schemes have benefits in their own right; they are not second-best substitutes for self-help groups. Befriendees feel that they have someone on whom they can rely, and who will be there for them. The befriender often feels more useful giving help to one particular person than acting in a group. Often the befriendee is more open at first in letter-writing and phone calls than they would be in a face-to-face meeting.

Such relationships can lead to many of the benefits described above for self-help groups. Whether such a scheme is generally successful is not known, as up until now it has not been monitored.

Penpal schemes are similar, exce¡ ι that, of cou.se, the relationship is more equal from the beginning. Participants advertise for sufferers with specific qualities, and therefore can communicate with the sort of person they require. Again, hov successful these schemes are is not known, as they have not been monitored.

Summary

Treating yourself by self-help, and being part of an organization of IBS sufferers, may make you feel a lot better, both psychologically and even physically. You may gain more confidence in yourself and your ability to cope, both with social situations and in relationships. You will have a lot more information, and so be in a better position to deal with medical practitioners. You will be able both to give and to receive emotional and social support; and other sufferers can help you through the bad times.

Group activities are likely to decrease depression, anxiety and stress and therefore have an indirect effect on symptoms, breaking the vicious cycle of symptoms leading to stress, leading to an aggrevation of symptoms. Although a self-help group cannot cure your IBS, it can have a positive impact on your life overall, and should be considered as part of the total treatment of Irritable Bowel Syndrome.

Appendix

This information given here is reproduced in good faith. The authors and publishers cannot be held responsible for any inaccuracies, nor do they recommend any products or services.

Useful General Books

C. P. Dancey and S. Backhouse, *Overcoming IBS* (London: Robinson, 1993)

V. Coleman, *Stress and Relaxation* (London: Hamlyn, 1993)

P. J. Donoghue and M. Siegel, *Sick and Tired of Feeling Sick and Tired: Living with Invisible Chronic Illness* (London: Norton, 1994)

R. Nicol, *Coping Successfully with Your Irritable Bowel* (London: Sheldon Press, 1989)

D. Potterton, *Herbal Remedies: IBS* (Foulsham, Berks, 1992)

M. Stewart and A. Stewart, *Beat IBS Through Diet* (London: Vermillion, 1994)

S. Trickett, *IBS and Diverticulosis: A Self-Help Plan* (London: Thorsons, 1990)

Watts, G., *IBS: A Practical Guide* (Cedar Press, 1990)

Also:

What Doctors Don't Tell You: a monthly newsletter covering thoroughly researched health topics. Available from 4 Wallace Road, London N1 2PG

Nutritional Treatments

Useful Addresses
Action Against Allergy (AAA), Greyhound House, 23–24 George St, Richmond, Surrey TW9 1JY

Institute for Optimum Nutrition, 5 Jerdan Place, London SW6 1BE

National Society for Research into Allergy, 26 Welwyn Road, Hinckley, Leics LE10 1JY

Register of Nutritional Therapists, Hatton Green, Warwick CV35 7LA

Society for Promotion of Nutritional Therapy, 2 Hampden Lodge, Hailsham Road, Heathfield, East Sussex TN21 8AE

Useful Books
J. Brostoff and L. Gamlin, *The Complete Guide to Food Allergy and Intolerance* (London: Bloomsbury, 1989)

Honor J. Campbell, *The Foodwatch Alternative Cookbook* (Bath: Ashgrove, 1988)

David Canter, Kay Canter and Daphne Swann, *The Cranks Recipe Book* (London: Grafton Books, 1982)

S. Davies and A. Stewart, *Nutritional Medicine* (London: Pan, 1987)

L. Galland, *Allergy Prevention for Kids* (London: Bloomsbury, 1989): contains some good information on nutrition generally, although written with children particularly in mind

Rachel Haigh, *The Neal's Yard Bakery Wholefood Cookbook* (London: Dorling Kindersley, 1986)

Hilda Cherry Hills, *Good Food, Gluten Free* (Connecticut: Keats, 1976): contains good material on important nutrients for people avoiding gluten

G. Jacobs, *Candida Albicans: Yeast and Your Health* (London: Optima, 1990)

Jack Santa Maria, *Greek Vegetarian Cookery* (London: Rider, 1984)

Suppliers of Special Diet Products

Berrydales, Berrydale House, 5 Lawn Rd, London NW3 2XS: suppliers of dairy-, gluten- and egg-free products

Biocare Ltd, 17 Pershore Road South, Birmingham B30 3EE: mail order suppliers of nutritional supplements

Cirrus Associates (South West), Little Hintock, Kington Magna, Gillingham, Dorset SP8 5EW: food and environmental consultancy; mail order suppliers of 'Arise' raising agent and other products

Green Farm Nutrition Centre, Burwash Common, East Sussex TN19 7LX: mail order suppliers of nutritional supplements

Foodwatch International Ltd, 9 Corporation Street, Taunton, Somerset TA1 4AJ: mail order suppliers of foods for special diets

Nutricia Dietary Products Ltd, 494–496 Honeypot Lane, Stanmore, Middx HA7 1JH: suppliers of gluten-free products

Sunnyvale Organic Breads and Cakes, Everfresh Natural Foods, Gatehouse Close, Aylesbury HP19 3DE: foods suitable for gluten-free, vegan and yeast-free diets

The Candida Shop, Natural Ways, Arfryn Caergeiliog, Anglesey, Gwynedd LL65 3NL: sells various products and advises on candida problems

Hypnotherapy

Physicians Practising Gut-Directed Hypnotherapy within the NHS
Dr P. J. Whorwell, BSc MD FRCP, Consultant Physician and Senior Lecturer in Medicine, Department of Medicine, Withington Hospital, Nell Lane, West Didsbury, Manchester M20 8LR

Dr P. Cann, FRCP, Consultant Physician and Gastroenterologist, Department of Medicine, Middlesbrough General Hospital, Ayresome Green Lane, Middlesbrough, Cleveland TS5 5AZ

Dr Alastair Forbes, BSc MD MRCP, Consultant Physician and Gastroenterologist, St Mark's Hospital, City Road, London EC1V 2PS

Dr I. Cobden, MD FRCP, Consultant Physician and Gastroenterologist, North Tyneside District Hospital, North Shields, Tyne and Wear NE29 0LR

The Register of Approved Gastrointestinal Psychotherapists and Hypnotherapists
For explanatory pamphlet and list of registered therapists in your area please send a large SAE to:

Elizabeth Taylor, Co-ordinator, 5 Stonefold, Rising Bridge, Accrington, Lancs BB5 2DP

Complementary Medicine

Useful Addresses (General)
Alternative Health Information Bureau, 12 Upper Station Road, Radlett, Herts WD7 8BX, tel./fax 01923 857670

British Complementary Medicine Association, Mental Health Unit, St Charles Hospital, Exmoor Street, London W10 6DZ, tel. 0181 964 1205

Institute of Complementary Medicine, PO Box 194, London

SE16 1QZ, tel. 0171 237 5165: advice on finding reputable practitioners

Chinese Medicine

British Acupuncture Association and Register, 34 Alderney Street, London SW1, tel. 0171 834 1012/6229). They will send you a list of their members. Their members are not allowed to advertise but you can find practitioners in the Yellow Pages. They advise looking for the designation MBAcA or FBAcA (Membership or Fellowship of the BAAR). All their full members are qualified in another form of medicine apart from acupuncture. Members can issue sickness certificates.

The British College of Acupuncture, 8 Hunter Street, London WC1N 1BN, tel. 0171 833 8164. They run a teaching clinic where treatment is available at reduced fees under the supervision of qualified practitioners.

International Register of Oriental Medicine (UK), 4 The Manor House, Colley Lane, Reigate, Surrey, RH2 9JW. Members are designated by the initials MIROM or IROM after their names.

An interesting book is Richard Lucas, *The Secrets of the Chinese Herbalists* (Wellingborough: Thorsons, 1978).

Homoeopathy

The British Homoeopathic Association, 27A Devonshire Street, London W1N 1RJ, tel. 0171 935 2163

The Royal London Homoeopathic Hospital, Great Ormond Street, London WC1N 3HR, tel. 0171 837 3091) (Homoeopathic prescriptions are available on the NHS.)

Herbalism

National Institute of Medical Herbalists, 9 Palace Gate, Exeter EX1 1JA, tel. 01392 426022

Naturopathy
General Council and Register of Naturopaths, Frazer House, 6 Netherhall Gardens, London NW3 5RR, tel. 0171 435 8728

British College of Naturopathy and Osteopathy, Frazer House, 6 Netherhall Gardens, London NW3 5RR, tel. 0171 435 7830

Reflexology
The British School of Reflexology, The Holistic Healing Centre, 92 Sheering Road, Old Harlow, Essex, CM17 0JW, tel. 01279 29060

International Federation of Reflexology, 51 Champion Close, Croydon, Surrey CR0 5SN, tel. 0181 680 9631

Colonic Irrigation
Colonic Irrigation Association, 50A Morrish Road, London SW2 4EG, tel. 0181 671 7136

Aromatherapy
The International Society of Professional Aromatherapists, Hinckley and District Hospital and Health Centre, The Annexe, Mount Road, Hinckley, Leics, LE10 1AG, tel. 01455 637987

The International Federation of Aromatherapists, Stamford House, 2-4, Chiswick High Road, London W4 1TH, tel. 0181 742 2605

Bach Flower Remedies
The Dr Edward Bach Healing Centre, Mount Vernon, Bakers Lane, Brightwell cum Sotwell, Wallingford, Oxon OX10 0PZ, tel. 01491 839489

Index